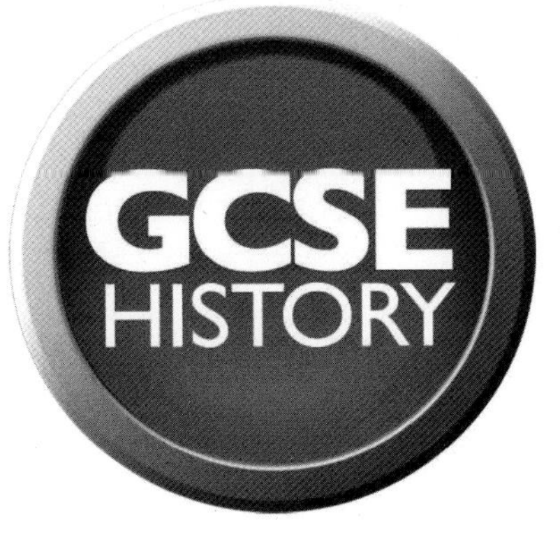

RAISING GRADES IN GCSE HISTORY

Medicine Through Time

Steve Waugh

Acknowledgements

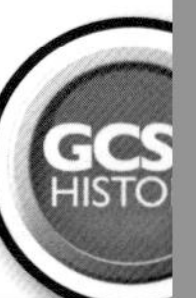

Editor: Joanne Mitchell
Layout artist: Book Matrix
Illustrations: Tony Randell
Cover design: Blayney Partnership
Cover image: Corbis

First published 2007 by Folens Limited.

Every effort has been made to contact copyright holders of material used in this publication. If any copyright holder has been overlooked, we should be pleased to make any necessary arrangements.

British Library Cataloguing in Publication Data. A catalogue record for this publication is available from the British Library.

ISBN 978 1 85008 226-2

Contents

Introduction

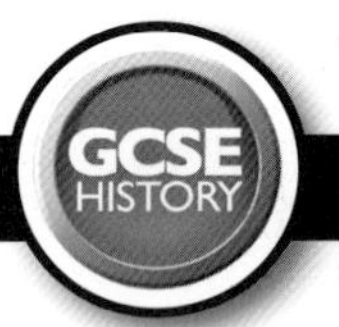

Raising Grades in GCSE History have been specifically written for teachers to use with students who may struggle with some of the skills and concepts needed for GCSE History. Each book in the series contains ten separate units covering the key developments within the topic of the book and developing the key skills needed for essay writing and interpretation skills for all of the GCSE specifications. Each unit has one or more photocopiable resource sheets and several activity sheets that provide an activity or activities to reinforce understanding, followed by activities which develop a particular skill, for example source inference questions. This allows the teacher to work in different ways. The tasks are differentiated throughout the book and offer all students the opportunity to expand their skills. By using photocopiable writing frames, students will be able to access historical information more easily and improve their essay and source skills in preparation for the examination.

The development of key skills

These include developing the ability to write causation, consequence, change, description and judgement essays. For sources and interpretations, students will practise inference, cross-referencing, utility, using a source and own knowledge and judging interpretations.

Objectives

These are the main skills and knowledge to be learned.

Prior knowledge

This refers to the minimum skills or knowledge required by students to complete the tasks. As a rule, students should have a reading comprehension age of 11–12 years and should be working at GCSE Levels 1 to 2. Some activity sheets are more challenging than others and teachers will need to select accordingly.

Links with GCSE specifications

All units link to at least two of the three main GCSE boards – AQA, Edexcel and OCR.

Background

This provides educational information for the teacher, expanding on historical details or giving further information about the unit.

Starter activity

Since the units can be taught as a lesson, a warm-up activity focusing on an aspect of the unit is suggested.

Resource sheets and activity sheets

The resource sheets, which are both visual and written, do not include tasks and can be used as stimuli for discussion. Related tasks are provided on the activity sheets.

Assessment sheet

At the end of each unit is an assessment sheet focusing on student progress. It can be used in different ways. A student can complete it as a self-assessment, while the teacher also completes one on each student's progress. They can then compare the two. This is useful where the teacher or classroom assistant is working with one student. Alternatively, students can work in pairs to carry out peer assessments and then compare the outcomes with each other. Starting from a simple base that students can manage, the assessment sheet allows the student to discuss their own progress, to consider different points of view and to discuss how they might improve, thus enabling the teacher to see the work from the student's perspective.

Plenary

The teacher can use the suggestions here to recap the main points covered or to reinforce a particular idea.

Other titles in the *Raising Grades in GCSE History* series:

- Russia 1900–1941
- Crime and punishment
- World War I
- International Relations 1919–1991
- USA 1919–1941
- Germany

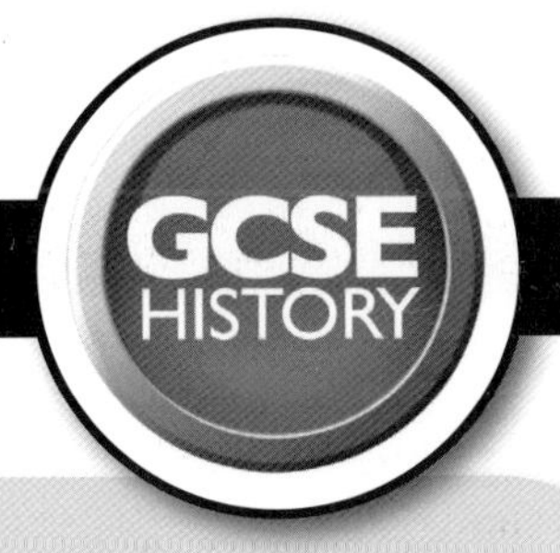

Medicine under the Greeks and Romans

Objectives

▸ Understand the key changes in medicine under the Greeks and Romans
▸ Complete a grid showing key changes
▸ Plan a change essay
▸ Be able to assess own progress

Prior knowledge

To achieve these objectives, students should have a reading age of 11–12 years and should have some understanding of chronology. They should also be able to use a writing grid.

Links with GCSE specifications

Edexcel: Medicine
AQA: Medicine and Public Health Through Time
OCR: Medicine Through Time

▸ Key study area
▸ Change essay

Background

The Egyptian civilisation lasted 3000 years. The Egyptians developed a form of writing that allowed them to keep records and write books, which meant they were able to pass on knowledge from generation to generation. For example, they 'mummified' dead bodies and, during the process, some internal organs were removed – they discovered the main internal organs. Records show that they had trained doctors who were also priests, but illness was thought to have spiritual causes. The Egyptians built large towns and so developed forms of public health for the first time. For example, a system of wells was constructed in the Nile Delta which provided fresh water for the pharaohs.

Starter activity

Students will need some understanding of the meaning of 'Medicine Through Time'. Provide each student with stick-it notes on which they can write two or three ideas about medicine. Stick their notes on the board to be used as a basis for a class discussion on the various features of medicine. You should narrow these down to five or six key areas, for example, doctors and nurses, surgery, hospitals and so on.

Resource sheets and activity sheets

Read through both resource sheets with the students and answer any questions they may have.

For 'Key changes under the Greeks and Romans', students could work in groups, with each group researching one key area of change. Alternatively, students could work in pairs, with one student completing the column on the Greeks and the other the column on the Romans. Continue with a whole class discussion on the most important change.

Enlarge 'Planning the change essay'. For activity sheets 'Change essay' and 'Planning the change essay', students should cut up the answer, arranging it into paragraphs to place on the planning grid. Hold a whole class discussion about the most important change.

Plenary

Divide the students into pairs for a game of 'history tennis'. Each student, in turn, should be asked a question about key changes under the Greeks or Romans. A correct answer means they score. The winner is the first student to win a tennis game.

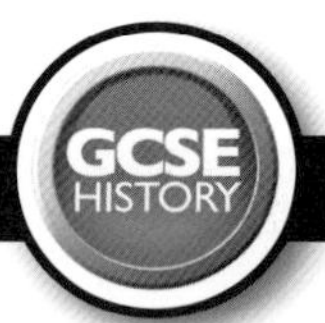

Medicine under the Greeks (1000–300 BCE)

The Greeks began to believe that disease had a natural cause. This meant that doctors started to look more closely at the body. However, dissection was not encouraged and surgery was still simple, for example, mending broken bones. In Alexandria, they did practise dissection and so learned more about anatomy.

In about 400 BCE, Hippocrates suggested that diseases have internal, personal, causes; they were not caused by gods or spirits. He said that the body contained four humours or fluids: black bile, yellow bile, blood and phlegm. Human beings became ill when these humours were unbalanced.

Hippocrates took care to observe and record each patient's symptoms. He said that people should lead simple, balanced lives in order to keep these humours in balance. He was the founder of the medical profession. The Hippocratic Oath (that a doctor will always try to save a patient and act only in the patient's interests, without fear or favour) is still taken by all doctors to this day.

From about 400 BCE, Hippocrates led the way with clinical observation and the Theory of the Four Humours: the first rational explanation of the cause of disease. Doctors trained in these beliefs were the first we recognise as doctors, not priests. This was the beginning of the medical profession.

Most Greeks lived in small towns on the edge of the sea. This meant that public health was not a problem.

At first, women were not allowed to train as doctors. One woman, Hagnodice, pretended to be a man and trained to be a doctor. She became popular with female patients. When it was discovered that Hagnodice was a woman, the law was changed to allow women who were not slaves to train as doctors. Many women became doctors and often went to work in the Roman Empire.

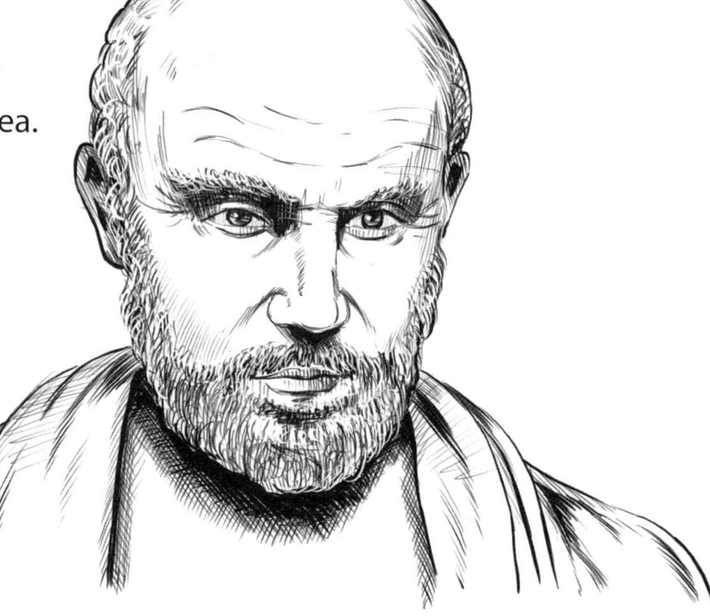

Hippocrates

The Greeks were the first people to realise that disease had natural causes. This developed from the ideas of Hippocrates. Although many people still believed diseases were caused by supernatural events, Hippocrates suggested ways in which people could try to avoid disease and practical methods of trying to cure themselves.

  Medicine Through Time

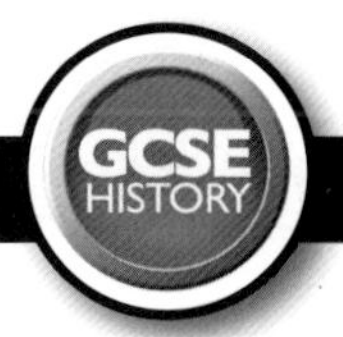

Medicine under the Romans (300 BCE–500 CE)

In the early centuries, the Romans believed in supernatural causes of disease. They believed that epidemic diseases were punishments from the gods. The work of Galen made many turn to more natural causes and remedies. After 300 CE, the Roman Empire was officially Christian and this further encouraged people to think that disease had natural causes. Before this date, the Romans appealed to their gods, chiefly Salus, the goddess of health.

Roman doctors were encouraged to improve their knowledge of anatomy. They established military hospitals for wounded soldiers. These gave many surgeons 'hands-on' experience and forced them to find ways of helping the wounded. They appear to have had opium to sedate patients and special cutting tools used for operations.

There were many doctors in the Roman Empire, most of whom were Greeks. Doctors such as Galen also treated the gladiators and gained a great deal of experience. Most trained doctors were men but the majority of care would still have been in the hands of wives and mothers.

The most important figure in Roman medicine was Claudius Galen. Galen was born in about 129 CE in Greece. He worked in Alexandria in Egypt, before coming to Rome. He took up the Theory of the Four Humours, wrote over 60 books – which were used by medical surgeons for the next 1500 years – and was the most famous doctor of the Roman world. He developed a system of treatments by opposites: treating imbalance in the four humours by giving something opposite to the humour that was in excess.

Galen

The Romans believed that personal cleanliness was very important. Every town and city had public baths. In Rome, there were dozens of baths and Romans spent up to two hours a day in them. They even conducted business there. The Romans also educated people to think that public health was important – '*Salus populi suprema lex esto*' (the health of the people is the highest law). Roman cities also had fresh water and drains. Canals and aqueducts were built to bring water to towns. Sewers were flushed through with rainwater; this kept them clean and stopped them blocking up.

Roman society was dominated by men; few women played important roles. Soranus, in the second century, wrote that there were trained female midwives in Rome. Midwives dealt with birth but they would also have had knowledge of how to deal with regular childhood ailments.

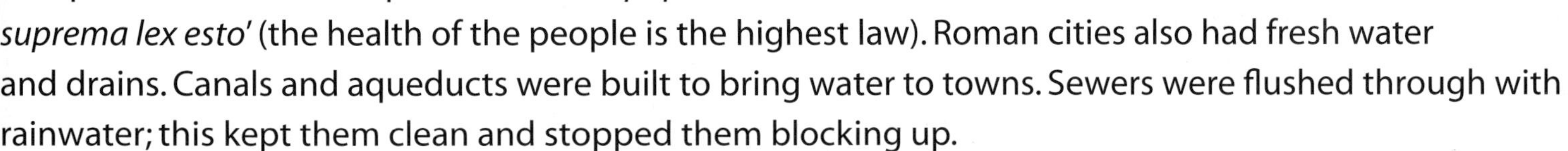

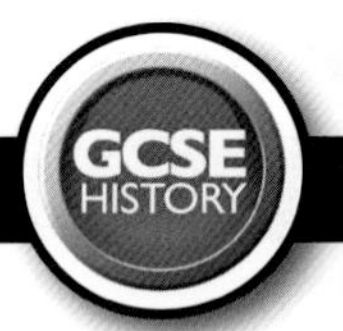

Key changes under the Greeks and Romans

Complete the chart below to summarise the key changes in medicine under the Greeks and Romans.
One has been done for you.

	Greeks	**Romans**
Key individuals		
Public health		
Doctors		
Women		
Causes of disease		At first, they believed in the supernatural but gradually many moved to natural causes.
Surgery		

What do you think was the most important change under the Greeks or Romans?

The most important change was ....

This was because ....

     Medicine Through Time

Change essay

In what ways were there changes in medicine under the Greeks and Romans?

Below is an answer to the above question. However, the student has mixed up what happened and has included information not relevant to this question and has not used paragraphs.

Using scissors, cut up the answer and re-arrange it in paragraphs in the right order on the next page, adding any important changes not mentioned. Remember to cross out any information not relevant to this question. Decide the most important change and explain it in the last row on 'Planning the change essay'.

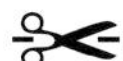

The work of Galen and Christian influence meant that more and more people in the Roman Empire began to believe that disease had natural causes. The Romans conquered Italy and most of Europe and built up a huge Empire. In about 400 BCE, Hippocrates suggested that diseases have internal, personal, causes; they were not caused by gods or spirits. He said that the body contains four humours or fluids: black bile, yellow bile, blood and phlegm. Human beings became ill when these humours were unbalanced. The Romans believed that personal cleanliness was very important. Every town and city had public baths. In Rome, there were dozens of baths and Romans spent up to two hours a day in them. The Romans also educated people to think that public health was important – '*Salus populi suprema lex esto*' (the health of the people is the highest law). Ancient Greece was not one country. The Greek people lived on the land and islands around the eastern Mediterranean. The most important figure in Roman medicine was Claudius Galen. Galen was born in about 129 CE in Greece. He worked in Alexandria in Egypt, before coming to Rome. He took up the Theory of the Four Humours, wrote over 60 books – which were used by medical surgeons for the next 1500 years – and was the most famous doctor of the Roman world. The Greeks began to believe that disease had a natural cause. This meant that doctors started to look more closely at the body. However, dissection was not encouraged and surgery was still simple, for example, mending broken bones. In Alexandria, they did practise dissection and so learnt more about anatomy. Roman doctors were encouraged to improve their knowledge of anatomy. They established military hospitals for wounded soldiers. These gave many surgeons 'hands-on' experience and forced them to find ways of helping the wounded. They appear to have had opium to sedate patients and special cutting tools used for operations.

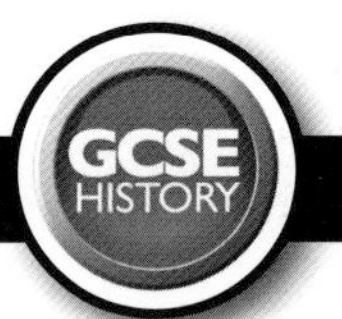

Planning the change essay

Arrange the cut-out answer from 'Change essay' in the boxes below.

Understanding of disease

Doctors and surgery

Key individuals

Public health

Women

Most important change:

Why?

     Medicine Through Time   © Folens (copiable page)

Assessment sheet – Medicine under the Greeks and Romans

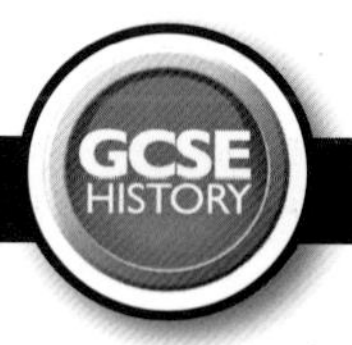

(✓) Tick the boxes to show what you know.

I know:

	know / yes	not sure / sometimes	don't know / no
why Hippocrates was important in medicine			
what was meant by the 'Four Humours'			
why Hagnodice pretended to be a man			
why Galen was important in medicine			
how the Romans improved public health			
why few women worked in medicine under the Romans			
how to complete a grid on change			
how to plan an essay on change			

I know best:

....

I need to work on (up to three targets):

....

....

....

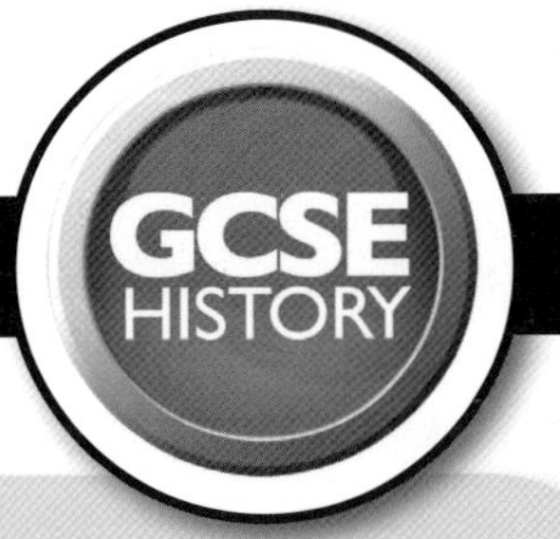

Medicine in Western Europe in the Middle Ages, 1066–1400

Objectives

‣ Understand the key features of medicine in the Middle Ages
‣ Complete a grid assessing progress
‣ Write a describe essay
‣ Be able to assess own progress

Prior knowledge

To achieve these objectives, students should have a reading age of 11–12 years and should have some understanding of chronology. They should also be able to use a writing grid.

Links with GCSE specifications

Edexcel: Medicine
AQA: Medicine and Public Health Through Time
OCR: Medicine Through Time

‣ Describe essay

Background

After the final collapse of the Roman Empire in the West in 476 CE, Europe experienced centuries of upheaval. This period of about 400 years has been called the 'Dark Ages' because there are few surviving records to tell us about the period. Probably in the 10th century, the famous medical school at Salerno in Italy was founded. The first universities appeared in the 12th century.

Starter activity

To improve their ability to describe precisely, divide the students into pairs. They should sit back to back. One student should describe the illustration in the centre of resource sheet 'The Black Death' to the other student, who should sketch it as precisely as possible. Carry out a peer assessment of how accurately reproduced the illustration is. Carry out a class discussion on the importance of precise description followed by interpretation of the illustration. What does the illustration reveal about medical beliefs in the Middle Ages?

Resource sheets and activity sheets

After reading the resource sheets 'Improvement or not?' and 'The Black Death', students could work in pairs with each group researching medicine in the Middle Ages, with one looking for improvement and the other for lack of progress to complete the table for activity sheet 'Was there improvement in the standard of medicine in the Middle Ages?'. This could be followed by a class discussion based on the rating line. The class could be divided into four groups, each of which researches and reports back on one feature of the Black Death.

Activity sheets 'Describe essay' and 'Writing your essay' practise the students' skills in precise description. Students could work in pairs when assessing the answer. Encourage feedback on the level and how it could be improved.

Plenary

Students could work in groups of four to summarise the main features of the Black Death using each of the following methods:

‣ bullet points;
‣ a sketch or storyboard;
‣ a mind map;
‣ a paragraph of less than 100 words.

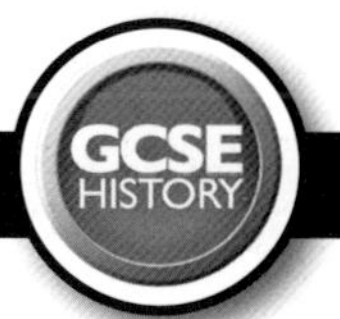

Improvement or not?

A group of students are discussing whether there was any improvement in medical knowledge and understanding in Western Europe in the Middle Ages.

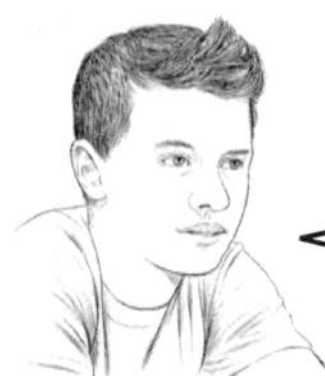

Andrew: I think there was some improvement because universities and medical schools were set up all over Europe which improved training.

Victoria: That is true, but treatment hardly changed and was still heavily influenced by the notion of the Four Humours. The theories of Galen were often combined with superstition to produce some strange cures.

Michael: Yes, theories of disease continued to be based largely on superstition. One example was hanging a dead magpie around the neck as a cure for toothache.

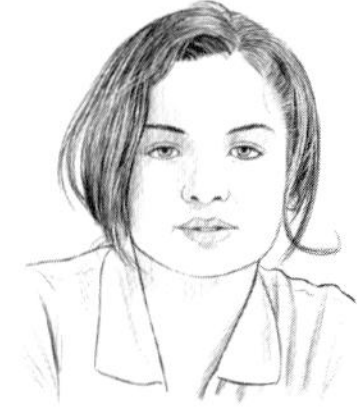

Rachel: Hang on. There was some progress. Many more hospitals were founded in Europe, many of which were attached to monasteries. London had four leper hospitals in the 14th century.

Victoria: It's no good having hospitals if doctors did not know how to treat patients. The most common remedy for virtually any illness was 'bleeding'. This actually caused considerable damage by causing anaemia, which means there are not enough red blood cells, or blood poisoning.

Peter: An increase in wars meant that surgeons had a lot more practice and gained a lot of practical experience.

Michael: That is true but their methods of treating wounds did not change. Limbs were amputated and the stump was cauterised with oil.

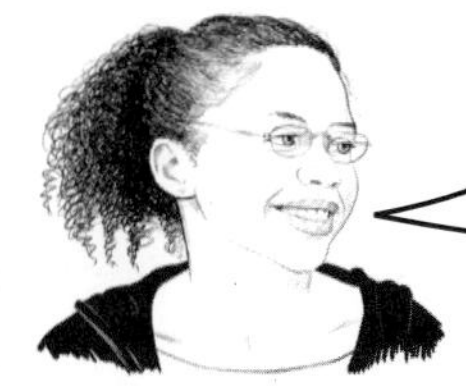

Jessica: There was some progress in surgery. One important surgeon was Roger of Salerno whose methods were based on the Greeks and Arabs.

Peter: Don't forget the new pharmacies that were set up, influenced by the Arabs, which sold herbs and medicines.

Victoria: Doctors still had only one form of diagnosis – urine analysis. They used pictures of the 21 shades of urine which had first been described in the 7th century.

The Black Death

What caused it?

The Black Death was what is known as 'bubonic plague'. The disease reached Britain around August 1348 and, by 1349, had spread throughout the country. We now know that the plague was a tiny germ, invisible except through a microscope, that lived in fleas which in turn lived on black rats. When the rats who had the plague died, the fleas moved onto humans who then caught the plague germ in their blood as soon as the flea bit them. The epidemic started in Asia and spread to Europe by ships carrying the infected rats.

Its symptoms

The plague passed rapidly from person to person and place to place. Someone could be feeling well in the morning and be dead by midday. Few people who caught it lived for more than three to four days. An Italian poet described its symptoms: 'In men and women alike it first showed itself by the appearance of swellings in the groin and armpits. Some grew as large as an apple or an egg. From these two parts of the body this deadly swelling soon began to spread in all directions. Then black spots began to appear.'

Why it spread

People could see it coming but did not know what to do to avoid it or what caused it. Most simply waited, hoping against hope that they and their families would survive. People at the time gave various reasons for the Black Death:

- Some people believed it was caused by poison caused by the Jews or cripples;

- Others blamed it on the position of the three great planets – Jupiter, Mars and Saturn;

- Many believed it was a punishment from God for all their sins.

Its effects

Those who thought the plague had been sent by God to punish their sins beat themselves to make up for their sins. They were known as flagellants. Between 1347 and 1349, the Black Death killed about one out of every three people living in Europe. It killed every sort of person, rich and poor alike. In some villages no one survived at all. In others, the number of people left was sometimes as few as half the original population. The fall in population meant there were not enough peasants left to work the land. That meant that the amount of money and food the lord received from his manor went down. However, the remaining peasants were able to demand higher wages.

 Medicine Through Time © Folens (copiable page)

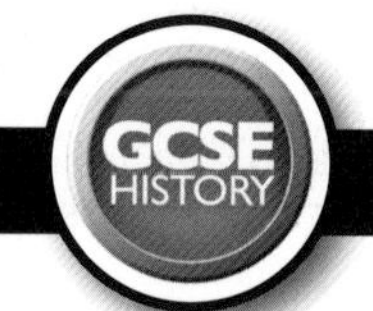

Was there improvement in the standard of medicine in the Middle Ages?

Using examples from the discussion on 'Improvement or not?', complete the table giving examples of progress or lack of progress in medicine in the Middle Ages. One example has been done for you.

Progress	Lack of progress
Opening of universities and medical schools.	

Now make a final judgement on the rating line.

Much improvement	Some improvement	No change	Some decline	Much decline

Overall, I believe that ....

....

This is because ....

....

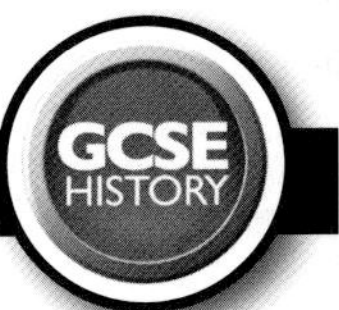

Describe essay

For a describe essay, it is important to ensure that:

▸ you describe key events and developments in the right order;

▸ you develop your descriptions with precise details.

Here is an example of how an answer could be marked.

Level 1	Simple or generalised answer. This might be a few short sentences which could apply to any event or person. There may be sentences which are not relevant to the question. Events are often in the wrong order.
Level 2	A more developed description of the key events which are in the correct sequence. It has more precise details. There is a paragraph on each key feature. It sticks to the dates of the question.

▸ Look at the sample answer below.

Describe the key features of the Black Death

The Black Death led to many deaths, with whole villages wiped out. In the Middle Ages, medical knowledge improved because of the opening of more universities. People who got the disease did not live longer than three days. Some people believed it was caused by the three great planets. It started with swellings in the groin and armpits. Then black spots appeared. Others believed it was a punishment from God. It was the bubonic plague. It was caused by fleas on rats. It killed about one out of every three people living in Europe. The Black Death was between 1348 and 1349.

Mark this answer and complete the grid. How could you improve this answer? Write your views in the third column.

Level	Reason	Target to improve

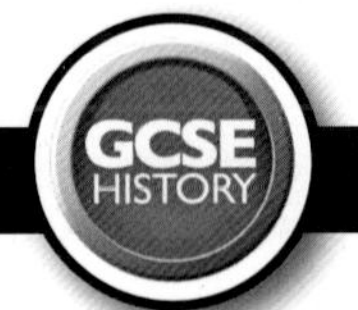

Writing your essay

Now write your own essay to describe the key features of the Black Death. Here is a writing grid to help you. You should:

▸ Give the feature;

▸ Describe it as precisely as you can.

Try to describe three key features, for example, its causes, symptoms and effects.

The first feature was ....

This ....

....

....

....

....

....

The second feature was ....

This ....

....

....

....

....

....

The third feature was ....

This ....

....

....

....

....

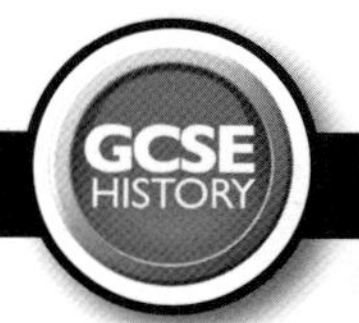

RAISING GRADES IN GCSE HISTORY

(✓) Tick the boxes to show what you know

I know:

	know / yes	not sure / sometimes	don't know / no
what the main cure was in the Middle Ages			
why there was increased medical knowledge			
what influenced most treatments			
what caused the Black Death			
why people did not understand it or stop it spreading			
the main symptoms of the Black Death			
how to describe key features			
how to assess a describe essay answer			

I know best:

....

I need to work on (up to three targets):

....

....

....

　　　Medicine Through Time　　　© Folens (copiable page)

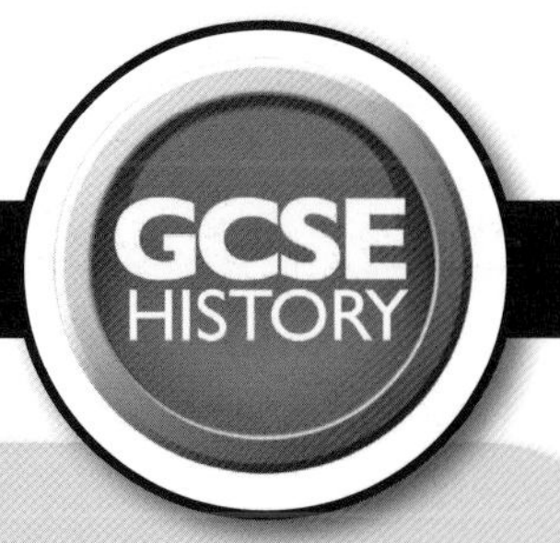

Changes in medicine, 1400–1700

Objectives

▸ Understand reasons why the Renaissance encouraged medical development
▸ Understand how to write a causation answer
▸ Be able to assess own progress

Prior knowledge

To achieve these objectives, students should have a reading age of 11–12 years and should have some understanding of causation. They should also be able to select simple information and use a writing frame.

Links with GCSE specifications

Edexcel: Medicine
AQA: Medicine and Public Health Through Time
OCR: Medicine Through Time

▸ Key study area
▸ Causation essay

Background

Renaissance means rebirth. The Renaissance was a period, roughly between 1400 and 1600, in which many forms of culture, especially drawing, painting, sculpture and literature, took huge steps forward. People at the time were inspired partly by looking back to Ancient Greece and Rome, and partly by trying out ideas which were new. The earliest centre of the Renaissance was Italy. It then spread to other parts of Europe, including Germany, the Netherlands, France and England.

Starter activity

Students should work in pairs. Show them the summary diagram of the Renaissance way of life on resource sheet 'The importance of the Renaissance'. Ask them to work out how and why the developments shown could help developments in medicine.

Resource sheets and activity sheets

For resource sheet 'The importance of the Renaissance', ask students, in groups, to research one of the reasons and to feed back to the whole class.

For resource sheet 'The impact of the scientific revolution on medicine', students could work in pairs and highlight, in different colours, reasons mentioned by the historian. Obtain feedback from the students on which were the most important factors in the Renaissance and the 'scientific revolution'.

'Why did the scientific revolution of the 17th century encourage progress in medicine?' should be done as a whole class activity. Explain different parts of the essay to the students including introduction, conclusion and reasons with explanation. Students could then add their own reasons, with explanations.

For 'Why did the Renaissance encourage progress in medicine?', students should write their own essay. Once completed, encourage volunteers to read out a paragraph of their essay to the class.

Plenary

As a group task and using a flow diagram, show the links between the various factors during the Renaissance and the scientific revolution. For example, printing brought wider publicity for art and sketches which showed exactly what the human body was like.

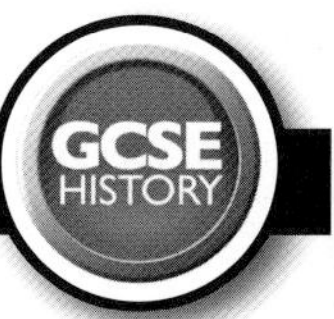

The importance of the Renaissance

The Renaissance encouraged progress in medicine for various reasons.

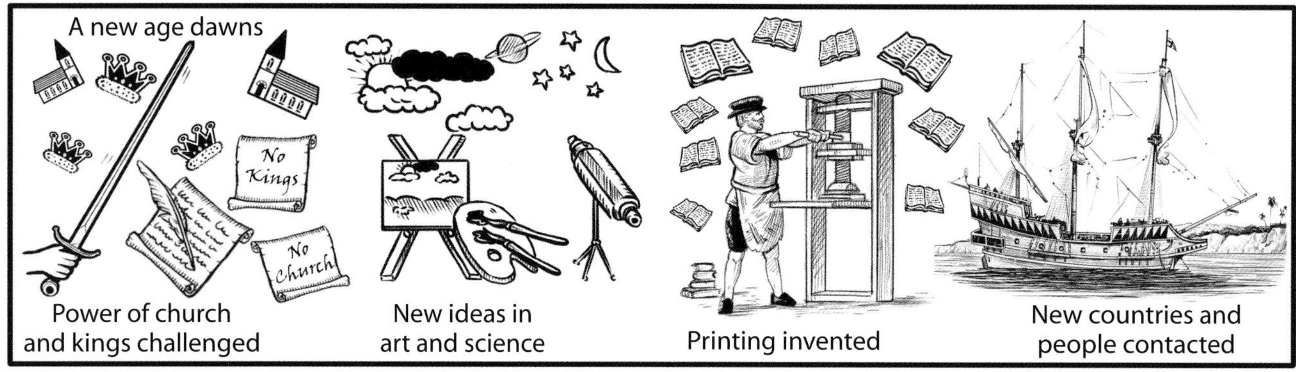

Art and the Renaissance

Artists helped the cause of medical knowledge a great deal. For example, Michelangelo's sculptures and paintings of the human figure were highly accurate and helped doctors to understand the way bodies are put together.

The Reformation

This was when many people changed to the Protestant religion. This reduced the influence of the Catholic Church. The Protestant churches encouraged people to do good works and many built hospitals and schools with the money they made.

Printing

In the Middle Ages, books were written by hand and took months, even years, to make. They were very expensive. All this was changed by Johannes Gutenberg who printed the first books in Europe in 1454. Many more people could now read the ideas of the Greeks and Romans, or the new ideas on medicine and religion. Soon doctors were questioning the old ideas about the human body.

Paracelsus

Paracelsus was typical of the new questioning of the human body. He was a town doctor and lecturer at Basel University. In 1527, he invited students, barber-surgeons and anyone who was interested to come to listen to him. He started his first lecture by burning a pile of books, including those written by Galen who he described as a liar and a fake.

The voyages of discovery

These opened up South America and brought many medical benefits. The best example was the import of quinine, an extract from cinchona bark. It provided effective treatment for malaria. It also encouraged doctors to question the symptoms of other diseases to see if other cures might be more readily available.

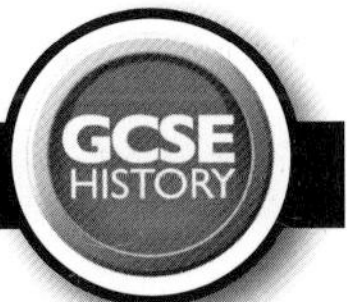

The impact of the scientific revolution on medicine

Here is an interview with an historian, about the part played by the Scientific Revolution in medicine.

Question: *What was meant by a 'scientific revolution'?*

Historian: These were scientific discoveries made in the different branches of medicine. For example, Galileo, who developed the telescope, and Descartes, who developed a new method of reasoning.

Question: *How did Descartes help medicine?*

Historian: His method of deductive reasoning perfectly fitted the needs of medicine. The doctor learned how to make deductions (educated guesses) from his patients' symptoms to diagnose what was wrong. A bit like Hippocrates.

Question: *What part was played by Galileo?*

Historian: His work on telescopes meant increased knowledge about lenses. This, in turn, encouraged men such as Anton van Leeuwenhoek to use them in an entirely new way – as microscopes to examine blood cells and bacteria.

Question: *How did developments in chemistry help medicine?*

Historian: An understanding of chemical processes led to a better understanding of reactions in the stomach.

Question: *What about physics? What benefits did that bring?*

Historian: Developments in the principles of mechanics helped people understand how muscles worked.

Question: *Were there any other important spin-offs for medicine?*

Historian: Yes, countries competed with each other in setting up academies of science. For example, in England we had the Royal Society. These academies greatly encouraged the spread of interest in new medical ideas and works. They also led to the publication of these new ideas.

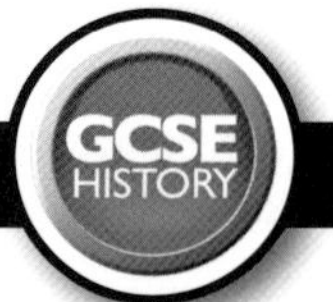

Why did the scientific revolution of the 17th century encourage progress in medicine?

Using the resource sheets 'The importance of the Renaissance' and 'The impact of the scientific revolution', write an essay explaining why the scientific revolution encouraged progress in medicine. Remember that essays beginning with 'why' are asking you to explain reasons.

Here is an example:

Introduction – here you have to explain key words in the question, for example, scientific revolution.

The scientific revolution was…

Now you have to give the reason.

The first reason was the influence of Descartes.

Now you have to explain the reason.

His method of deductive reasoning perfectly fitted the needs of medicine. The doctor learned how to make deductions (educated guesses) from his patients' symptoms to diagnose what was wrong. A bit like Hippocrates.

Now have a go yourself. Try to write two more reasons. Here is a writing grid to help you.

Another reason was

This

A third reason was

This

Now write a conclusion in which you explain which you think was the main reason.

Overall (begin with this word), I think the main reason was

This was because

     Medicine Through Time   © Folens (copiable page)

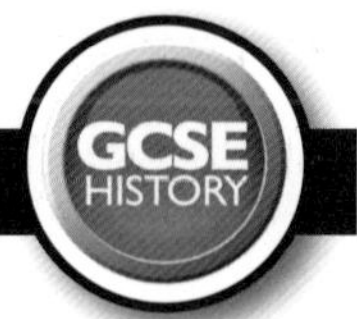

Why did the Renaissance encourage progress in medicine?

Have a go at writing an essay to explain why the Renaissance encouraged progress in medicine. Use highlighters:

▶ Red for the reason;
▶ Green for the explanation.

Introduction
The Renaissance was ....

....

Reasons
The first reason why the Renaissance encouraged progress in medicine was ....

....

This was ....

....

....

Another reason was ....

....

This was ....

....

....

A final reason was ....

....

This was ....

....

Conclusion
Overall, the most important reason was ....

....

This was because ....

....

Assessment sheet – Changes in medicine, 1400–1700

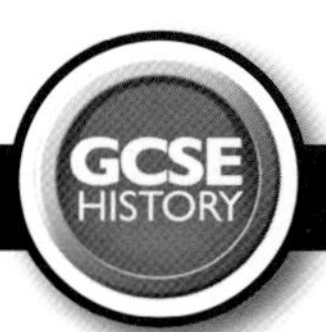

(✓) Tick the boxes to show what you know.

I know:

	know / yes	not sure / sometimes	don't know / no
what is meant by the Renaissance			
why printing helped medicine			
why the Reformation helped medicine			
the importance of Paracelsus			
how medicine was helped by Descartes			
what was meant by the 'scientific revolution'			
how to explain reasons			

I know best:

....

I need to work on (up to three targets):

....

....

....

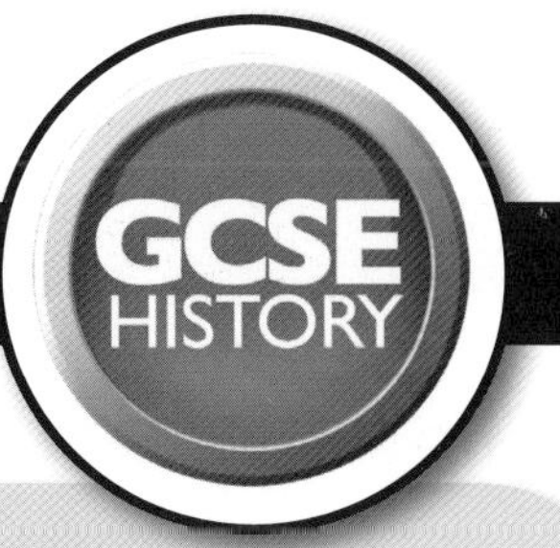

The importance of individuals in developments in medicine, 1400–1700

Objectives

▸ Understand the part played by individuals in the development of medicine
▸ Decide which factors influenced the work of the individual
▸ Understand how to write an essay on the importance of individuals
▸ Be able to assess own progress

Prior knowledge

To achieve these objectives, students should have a reading age of 11–12 years and should have some understanding of causation. They should also be able to select simple information and use a writing frame.

Links with GCSE specifications

Edexcel: Medicine
AQA: Medicine and Public Health Through Time
OCR: Medicine Through Time

▸ Key study area
▸ Essay on the contribution of individuals

Background

The Renaissance and Reformation provided an environment in which traditional ideas and practices were questioned. This, in turn, encouraged change. Medicine was no exception and several key individuals challenged the ideas of Galen and introduced important medical innovation – notably Andreas Vesalius, Ambroise Paré, William Harvey and Thomas Sydenham. Their changes, however, were not always universally accepted by medical practitioners of the time.

Starter activity

Brainstorm with the class the important individuals in medicine before 1400. Suggestions could be Hippocrates and Galen. Why were they important?

Resource sheets and activity sheets

Students could be divided into groups of four and asked to research all four individuals on resource sheets 'Vesalius and Paré and 'Harvey and Sydenham' and feed back to the whole group. The group could then complete the grid on activity sheet 'Chance and medicine' on factors which influenced each individual, and rank order the four men. This could be followed by a whole class discussion and vote on the rank order.

For 'Essay on the importance of individuals', students should each choose one of the four individuals listed and answer the two-part essay question. Obtain feedback from the students on their two-part answers.

'Essay on Paré' relates to 'Essay on the importance of individuals' and could be done as a paired activity. Students are required to put the parts of an essay answer in order.

Plenary

Divide the class into four groups. Each group has to:
▸ fully research one of the four individuals;
▸ set three or four questions on a second individual;
▸ choose a volunteer from each group to be 'hot seated'.
Each volunteer should be 'hot seated' and asked the three or four questions set by another group.

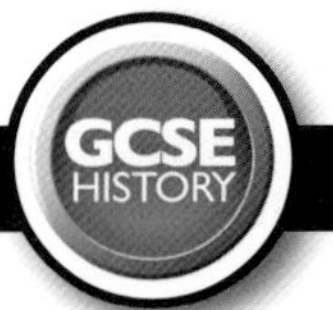

Vesalius and Paré

	Andreas Vesalius (1514–64)	**Ambroise Paré (1510–90)**
Background	He studied medicine in Paris and Italy and became Professor of Surgery at Padua in Italy.	In 1523, he went to Paris to train as a barber-surgeon. From 1536, he worked as an army surgeon.
Influences	As a student, he met artists who were studying skeletons and dissecting bodies to make their paintings more realistic. The decline of the Catholic Church meant that he was able to dissect bodies.	Over the previous 200 years, the use of guns in battles had increased. This led to a great number of casualties and different types of wounds. This, in turn, gave surgeons even more opportunity to practise, but no treatments worked.
Changes	He taught anatomy by doing his own dissections, normally done by assistants. He published drawings of these dissections. This led him to question the findings of Galen and show that he had made errors. In 1543, he published *On the Fabric of the Human Body* – a book on anatomy with drawings by first-class artists.	The usual treatment for gunshot wounds was to chop off damaged limbs and dip the stump in boiling oil. Paré ran out of oil and made up a treatment from turpentine, oil of roses and egg yolks. He also began to tie the arteries with silk thread. This stopped the patient bleeding to death. In 1585, he wrote in French *The Apology and Treatise of Ambroise Paré* describing his discoveries.
Importance	His work was accurate and printed and therefore available for training doctors. He proved that Galen had made mistakes about the nature of the human body and key organs. This encouraged other people to find out more. Vesalius also developed a new way of teaching – public dissection backed up by pictures.	His treatments worked and many soldiers survived. He understood how to test a theory to see if it worked. This is at the heart of modern scientific thinking. He made public his new ideas and methods so that other doctors could learn from them. His book was widely read.

 Medicine Through Time

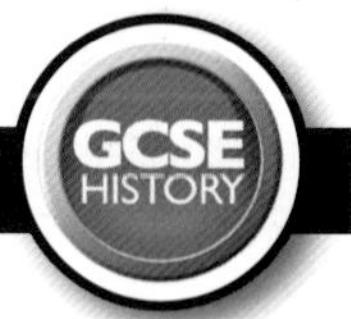

Harvey and Sydenham

	William Harvey (1578–1657)	**Thomas Sydenham (1624–89)**
Background	He studied medicine at Padua. Afterwards, he worked in London as a doctor and a teacher of anatomy. He was doctor to James I.	He studied at Oxford and Montpellier in France. He fought on Cromwell's side during the English Civil War and later became a doctor.
Influences	He was educated at Padua where he learned to question medical knowledge. He also grew up in a time when pumps were beginning to be used. He began to compare the heart to a pump.	Sydenham was influenced by the 'scientific revolution' of the time, particularly the method of careful observation and recording. He had read widely, especially the work of Harvey.
Changes	Until Harvey, doctors followed Galen's belief that blood moved through the heart by passing through the central wall. Harvey showed that blood was pumped by the heart around the body and re-used and moved from the heart to the lungs. The veins, arteries and valves made a one-way system through which blood passed.	He was a careful observer and recorded his observations in great detail in his main work, *Medical Observations*, in 1675. These descriptions included cholera, dysentery and measles. He considered there were two types of symptom: 'essential symptoms' from outside the body and 'accidental symptoms' from inside – in the form of the body's resistance.
Importance	Harvey published his findings in *An Anatomical Treatise on the Motion of the Heart and Blood*. He encouraged others to question medical ideas, especially those of Galen. However, many doctors did not accept Harvey's findings and continued to use bleeding as treatment.	He made no original discovery and accepted some old ideas, for example, diseases caused by foul airs or 'miasmas'. However, he established a new tradition of clinical observation. One of his followers, Walter Harris, applied Sydenham's techniques of observation to produce a book on the diseases of infants.

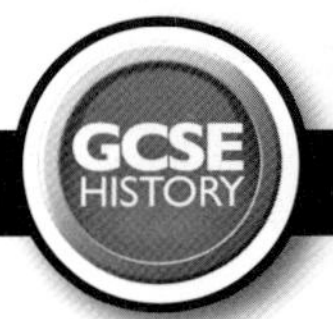

Chance and medicine

How did the four individuals make their contribution to medicine? Complete the following grid with a brief explanation of each choice. You may use all three columns for one individual. One example has been done for you.

	Chance	Influence others	Own work/publicity
Vesalius			
Paré	He ran out of boiling oil and had to use whatever materials were at hand.		
Harvey			
Sydenham			

Who made the most important contribution? Put your four individuals in order of importance on the diamond ranking below with the most important at the top and the least important at the bottom. Give an explanation for the first and last choices.

   Medicine Through Time   © Folens (copiable page)

Essay on the importance of individuals

Individuals have made important contributions to the development of medicine.
Choose **one** of the following individuals to write about: Vesalius, Paré, Harvey or Sydenham.

(a)   Explain the contribution he made to the development of medicine.

This part is asking you to explain any important changes brought about by the individual.

_________________________ made an important contribution because he ....

....

....

....

(b)   Was individual brilliance the only reason why he was able to make an important contribution to the development of medicine?

For this part you have to explain:
▸   the background/qualities of the individual;
▸   at least one other reason for his contribution.

Individual brilliance was important because _________________ ....

....

....

....

However, there was another reason which was ....

....

....

....

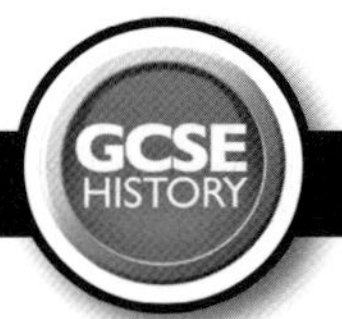

Essay on Paré

A student has been given the same essay as on 'Essay on the importance of individuals' and has chosen to write about Paré. However, the answer is badly organized. Read the following statements and put them in the right order for parts (a) and (b) as explained on 'Essay on the importance of individuals'.

1. Paré's contribution was also due to good luck. He was treating a gunshot wound when he ran out of boiling oil and had to use what was readily at hand.

2. Paré discovered that wounds healed more quickly if boiling oil was not used. Instead, he applied simple bandages. He also tied the ends of arteries with silk thread.

3. In 1585, he wrote in French *The Apology and Treatise*, describing his discoveries and enabling others to find out about his discoveries.

4. Paré used turpentine, oil of roses and egg yolks.

5. Paré made an important contribution to the treatment of wounds. Before Paré, wounds were treated by pouring boiling oil onto them. They stopped a wound bleeding by sealing it with a red-hot iron. This was known as cauterizing.

6. His contribution was partly due to his own brilliance. Although he had only trained as an inferior barber-surgeon, he joined the French army and was able to use this position to treat a great number of gunshot wounds.

(a)	
(b)	

Assessment sheet – The importance of individuals in developments in medicine, 1400–1700

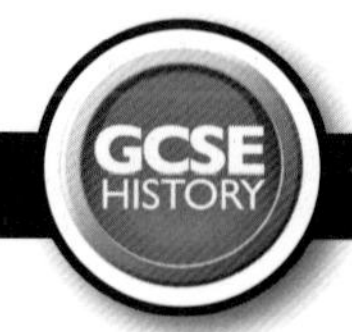

(✓) Tick the boxes to show what you know.

I know:

	know / yes	not sure / sometimes	don't know / no
why Vesalius is important in medicine			
how Paré changed the treatment of wounds			
what Harvey discovered about the circulation of blood			
how all three publicised their findings			
what contribution was made by Sydenham			
how to rank order individuals			
how to write a two-part essay answer			

I know best:

....

I need to work on (up to three targets):

....

....

....

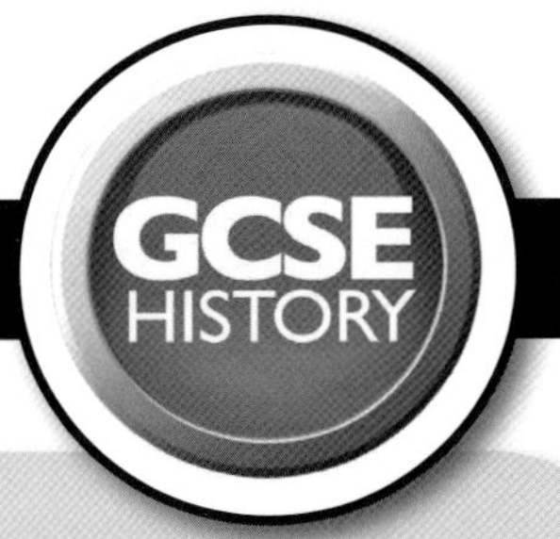

Changes in surgery, 1800–1900

Objectives

- Understand the developments in surgery in the 19th century
- Be able to complete a Venn diagram
- Understand how to write a judgement essay
- Be able to assess own progress

Prior knowledge

To achieve these objectives, students should have a reading age of 11–12 years and should have some understanding of causation. They should also be able to select simple information and use a writing frame.

Links with GCSE specifications

Edexcel: Medicine
AQA: Medicine and Public Health Through Time
OCR: Medicine Through Time

- Key study area
- Judgement essay

Background

There were many problems with surgery at the beginning of the 19th century. Operating theatres would have been unrecognisable to us today. They were rarely swept or cleaned and were often called slaughterhouses. Surgeons wore old coats which were rarely washed and never wore protective gloves. There were no anaesthetics so patients suffered awful pain. This meant that a surgeon had to act very quickly to prevent the patient dying of shock. Amputation of legs and arms was often done in under a minute. The absence of sterile conditions very often led to infection and complications. The most common were septicaemia (blood poisoning) and gangrene.

Starter activity

In pairs, students should study the cartoon on resource sheet 'The development of anaesthetics' and write down at least three problems with surgery. Give feedback and hold a whole class discussion of the main problems, which could include pain, infection and the loss of blood.

Resource sheets and activity sheets

Using the information given on the resource sheets 'The development of anaesthetics' and 'The work of Joseph Lister' and also the sources on the activity sheet 'Opposition to the changes', students could work in pairs. One student could research the key developments made by Simpson and Lister and the other the extent of opposition.

For 'Opposition to the changes', students should read the sources and then complete the table. One source could be done as a whole class activity. The activity could lead on to a whole class discussion on the reasons for the opposition. How justified was it? What effect did it have on progress?

Students should be able to complete 'The importance of changes' individually by reading each statement and relating it to a part of the Venn diagram.

The teacher should carefully explain the judgement essay for 'What made the greater contribution to surgery in the 19th century, anaesthetics or antiseptics?', stressing that activity sheets 'Opposition to the changes' and 'Importance of changes' will help with the second part of the essay.

Plenary

You could write up the following account and ask students to find the errors and replace them with the correct answers. A student has been asked to revise the key developments in surgery in the 19th century for a test. Here is their answer:

In 1846, Sir Humphrey Davy experimented with the use of ether as an anaesthetic. Four years later, Joseph Simpson, who was a dentist, accidentally discovered chloroform. There was much opposition to it but it became widely accepted when it was used on Queen Elizabeth I. James Lister played an important role in the development of antiseptics. He had seen the use of sulphuric acid in sewers and applied this to surgery.

Has the student revised thoroughly?

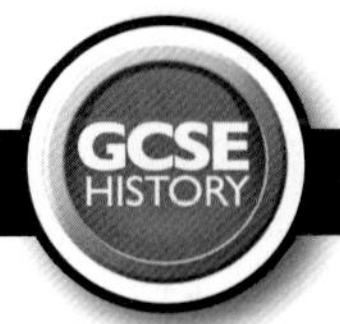

The development of anaesthetics

There were three main problems with surgery in the 19th century.

- Pain. This was tackled by anaesthetics.
- Infection. This was tackled by the development of antiseptics.
- Loss of blood. This was not tackled in the 19th century.

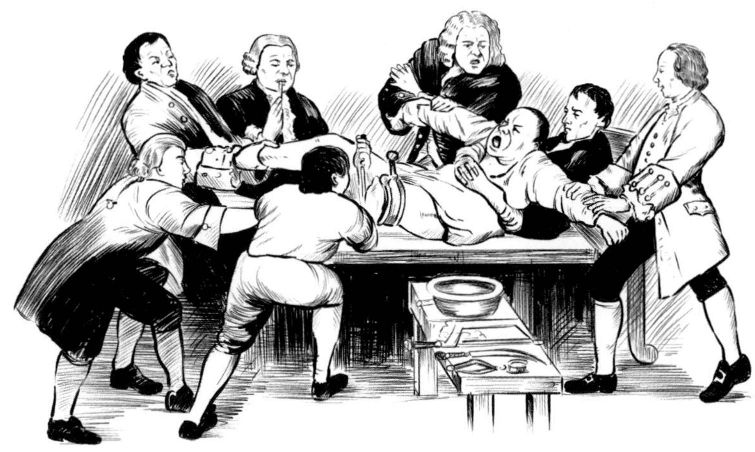

Anaesthetics

Date	Invention	Importance
1799	Sir Humphrey Davy discovered laughing gas (nitrous oxide).	He did not publish his findings very well so the discovery was not taken up.
1845	Horace Wells, an American dentist, used nitrous oxide on several patients.	It worked well at first but then one of his patients died.
1846	J R Liston used ether on a man having a leg amputated.	Queen Victoria used it for the birth of her eighth child in 1853. However, ether could catch fire and made patients cough a lot.
1847	James Simpson was Professor of Midwifery at Edinburgh University. Simpson and a few colleagues inhaled some chemicals and were all 'under the table' in a minute or two. Simpson realised that he had discovered chloroform, a powerful anaesthetic. He soon started using it to relieve women's labour pains. In 1857, Queen Victoria publicly praised the use of chloroform. It meant that surgeons could take more time over their operations and patients no longer had to be held down.	He wrote articles about its discovery and other surgeons began to use it in their operations. However, there was powerful opposition to the use of chloroform and anaesthetics. Many in the medical profession argued that it was a new and untested gas and no one was sure of its long-term effects. There were early deaths from its use. There were also religious arguments. Some people were particularly opposed to the idea of easing pain in childbirth, believing that this was unnatural.

 Medicine Through Time

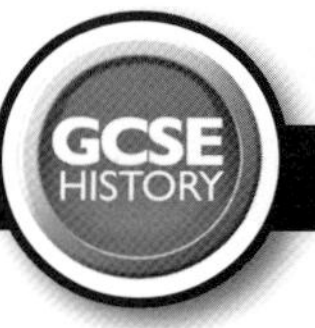

The work of Joseph Lister

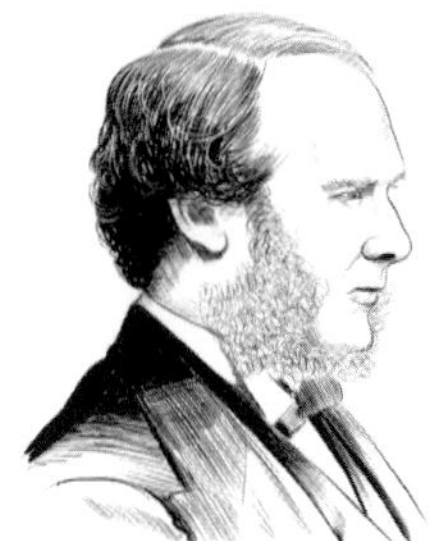

Lister was one of the outstanding surgeons of the 19th century. He had researched gangrene and infection and had a keen interest in the application of science to medicine. He read the work of Pasteur on germ theory, published in 1861.

Carbolic spray

Lister had seen carbolic spray used to treat sewage. After experiments, he found that a thin mist of carbolic acid sprayed over the wound during surgery reduced infection. This was called antiseptic as it killed 'sepsis' germs. By following this with careful bandaging, the wound would heal and not develop gangrene. Lister also tried to ensure that everything used in the operating theatre was

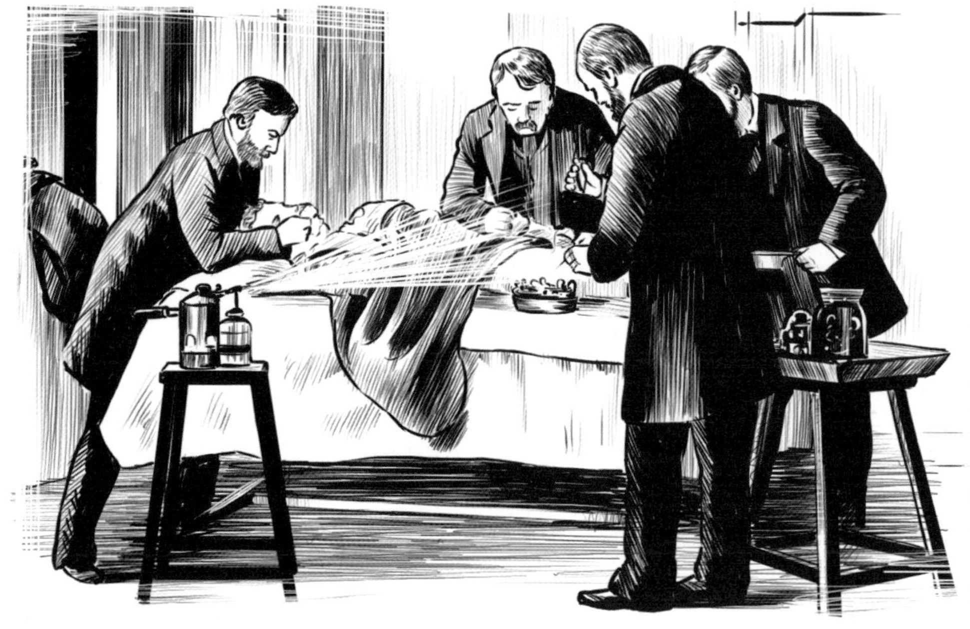

cleaned with carbolic acid to prevent the spread of germs. This included the surgeon's hands, the knives and the patient. Far fewer patients died because of infection.

Opposition to antiseptics

There was much opposition to Lister's methods.

- Lister was seen as a fanatic. His carbolic spray, which soaked the operating theatre, seemed very extreme. It cracked the surgeon's skin and made everything smell.
- The new precautions caused extra work, especially for the nurses and surgeons, and made operations more expensive.
- Surgeons believed that speed was essential in operations due to the problem of bleeding. Lister's methods seemed to slow operations down.

How did Lister change surgery?

In 1878, Koch found the bacterium which caused septicaemia. In the 1890s, he showed that the pus from patients' wounds was caused by germs on the surgeons' hands. This gave a great boost to Lister's ideas. By the 1890s, his antiseptic methods became aseptic surgery which meant removing all possible germs from the operating theatre. All operating theatres were rigorously cleaned and, from 1887, all instruments were steam-sterilised. Seven years later, rubber gloves were used for the first time.

Medicine Through Time

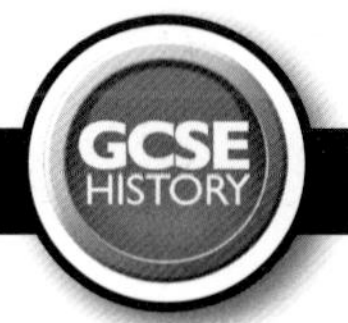

Opposition to the changes

Read the following sources.

Source A: From a medical journal.

> The infliction of pain has been invented by the Almighty God. Pain may be considered a blessing of the Gospel, and being blessed admits to being made either well or ill.

Source B: From a doctor.

> Anaesthetics are a most unnatural practice. The pain and sorrow of child labour improve the religious character of women. The Bible says that women should suffer pain during childbirth.

Source C: An Army Chief of Medical Staff.

> The smart use of the knife is a powerful stimulant and it is much better to hear a man bawl lustily than to see him sink silently into the grave.

Source D: From a doctor who worked with Lister.

> Among other things, it was difficult to convince surgeons that tiny objects of less than 0.001 mm in diameter could be the cause of the septic disease. The surgeons of the day were interested in keeping up their anatomy and increasing the number of operations. Minute germs seemed far removed from practical work.

Source E: From another doctor who worked with Lister.

> The nurses resented the extra work antiseptics gave them, such as the endless washing of basins and mackintoshes. One of the surgeons at St Bartholomew's could always raise a laugh by telling anyone in the room to shut the door quickly in case a microbe came in.

Place the source letter in the appropriate category in the table. Some may appear in more than one category.

	Religion/nature	**Medical profession**
Anaesthetics		
Antiseptics		

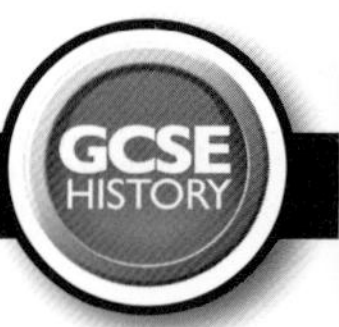

The importance of changes

The following statements explain the importance of the changes in surgery in the 19th century. Place each statement, by writing its number, in one part of the Venn diagram below.

1. The use of antiseptics had a dramatic effect, greatly reducing the number of deaths from gangrene and food poisoning.

2. When anaesthetics were safely and successfully used at the birth of Queen Victoria's son, Leopold, a lot of criticism of Simpson's chloroform stopped.

3. The death rate in 1873 before the introduction of antiseptics was 59.2%. The death rate after its introduction was 4%.

4. Lister's work was the beginning of modern surgery. Operations could now be done safely with surgeons working deep inside the body.

5. Anaesthetics and antiseptics together ensured that operations could be carried out much more gradually and with far less risk to the patient.

6. Chloroform meant that there was no longer the need to complete an operation within a few minutes. Instead of simply amputating the limbs, the surgeon could enter the abdominal and chest cavities.

7. Simpson and Lister both contributed greatly to surgery in the 19th century, ensuring that operations had a much greater chance of success.

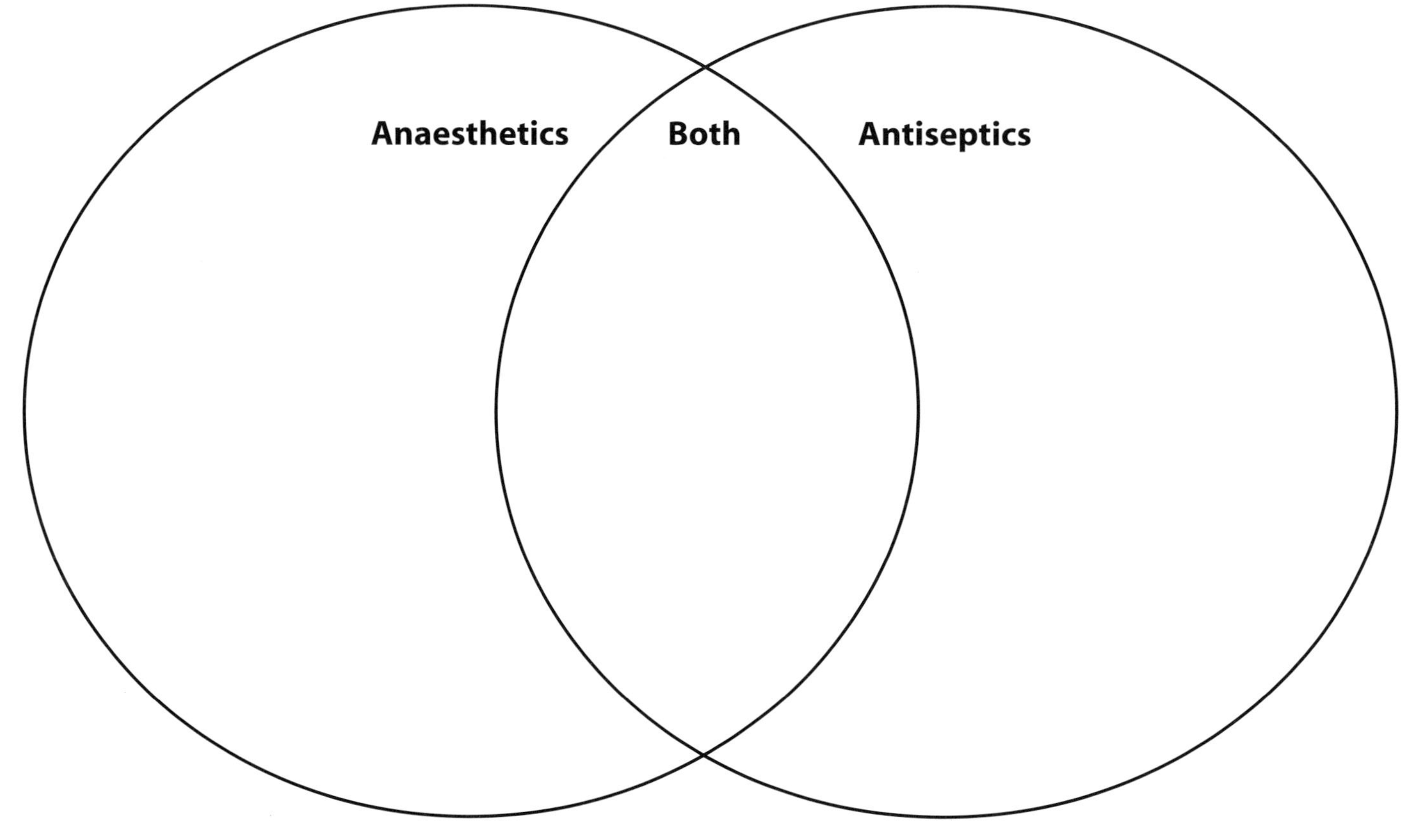

     Medicine Through Time

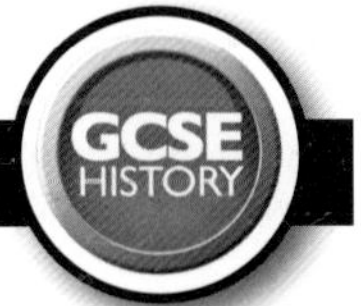

What made the greater contribution to surgery in the 19th century, anaesthetics or antiseptics?

This essay is asking you to give your judgement on which did more to improve surgery in the 19th century. Use 'Opposition to the changes' and 'The importance of changes' to help you. You should:

- explain the importance of each factor in turn;
- explain the limitations of each – especially the opposition;
- make a final judgement on which was the more important. Explain your judgement. You can decide that they were equally important as long as you give an explanation.

Here is the first half of the essay.

The development of anaesthetics was important because it meant that there was no longer the need to complete an operation within a few minutes. Instead of simply amputating the limbs, the surgeon could enter the abdominal and chest cavities. When anaesthetics were safely and successfully used at the birth of Queen Victoria's son, Leopold, chloroform, which had been developed by James Simpson, was widely used.

However, its contribution was delayed due to widespread opposition. Many in the medical profession argued that it was a new and untested gas and no one was sure of its long-term effects. There were early deaths from its use. There were also religious arguments. Some people were particularly opposed to the idea of easing pain in childbirth, believing that this was unnatural.

Now write the rest of the essay.

Antiseptics were important because ....

....

....

....

However, there was widespread opposition from ....

....

....

....

Overall, I believe (your final judgement) ....

....

....

....

Assessment sheet – Changes in surgery, 1800–1900

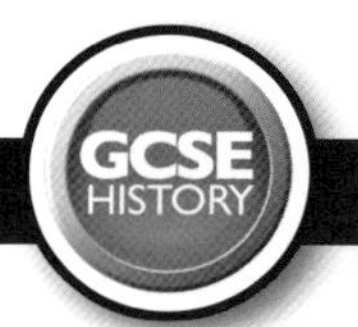

(✓) Tick the boxes to show what you know

I know:	know / yes	not sure / sometimes	don't know / no
why surgery was a problem in 1800			
how chloroform was developed			
why there was opposition to chloroform			
what part Queen Victoria played in the development of anaesthetics			
why Lister used carbolic acid			
how Lister's methods changed surgery			
why there was opposition to Lister's methods			
how to complete a Venn diagram			
how to write a judgement essay			

I know best:

....

I need to work on (up to three targets):

....

....

   Medicine Through Time   © Folens (copiable page)

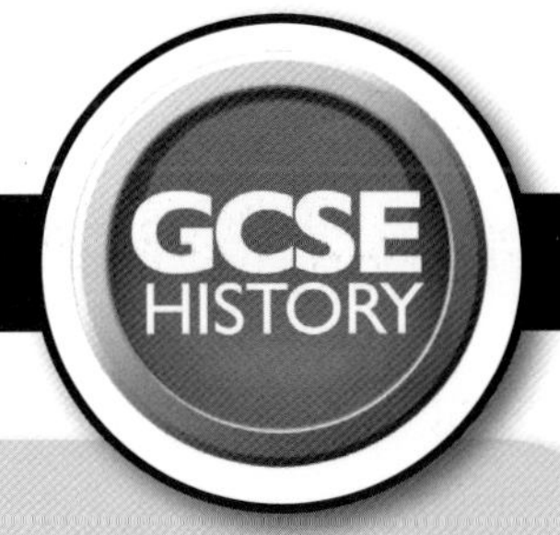

Changes in nursing in the 19th century

Objectives

- Understand the key changes in nursing in the 19th century
- Compare two illustrations
- Understand how to make inferences from a source
- Be able to assess own progress

Prior knowledge

To achieve these objectives, students should have a reading age of 11–12 years and should have some understanding of source skills. They should also be able to comprehend and interpret written sources.

Links with GCSE specifications

Edexcel: Medicine
AQA: Medicine and Public Health Through Time
OCR: Medicine Through Time

- Key study area
- Source inference skills

Background

The reputation of nursing in the early 19th century was very bad. Most nurses were untrained and poorly paid. They were little better than cleaners and were given little or no medical training. Women, in general, were regarded as second-class citizens. Indeed, women from a middle-class background, such as Florence Nightingale, were expected to marry and have children, not pursue a career. Those who did not marry could possibly work as a governess but not in the medical profession. Florence Nightingale broke the mould and at the same time brought great changes to nursing, helping to transform it into a serious, well-trained profession.

Starter activity

To encourage an understanding of inferences or messages from sources, ask the students to make inferences about their teacher. You could use a bag with personal items, such as a football programme, which give messages about the interest of the teacher. Explain how we also get messages from body language. Put the students in pairs. One student should use body language to give the other student a message.

Resource sheets and activity sheets

For resource sheets 'The work of Florence Nightingale' and 'Improvements in nursing', students could work in groups and research Florence Nightingale's early life and career. They could be asked to answer the question 'How did she break the mould or stereotype of middle-class 19th-century women?'

For activity sheet 'Improvements in hospitals', students could work in pairs to identify the changes between the two illustrations. Students may need more guidance on writing an obituary. Read out an example of an obituary to the class.

Explain the inferences on 'Inferences'. Obtain feedback from the students on their own inferences. Students could underline parts of the sources which show an inference.

For 'Assessing inferences', ensure that the students set a target for improvement for the candidate who has written a level 1 answer.

Plenary

Students could be divided into groups. Each group should consider how one of the following would react to Florence Nightingale's work in Scutari and feed back to the whole class, possibly in a role-play exercise:

- a middle-class man;
- a middle-class woman;
- a nurse;
- a male doctor.

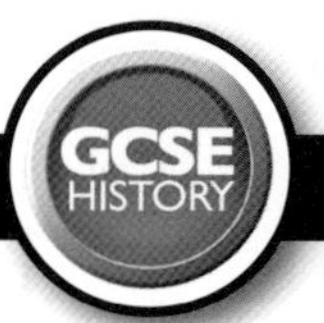

The work of Florence Nightingale

Nursing before Florence

Many of the nurses were badly paid, untrained, poorly educated and even drunken. Indeed, nurses were seen as no better than cleaners and were paid less than factory workers. They slept in the wards and often used part of their wages to buy gin.

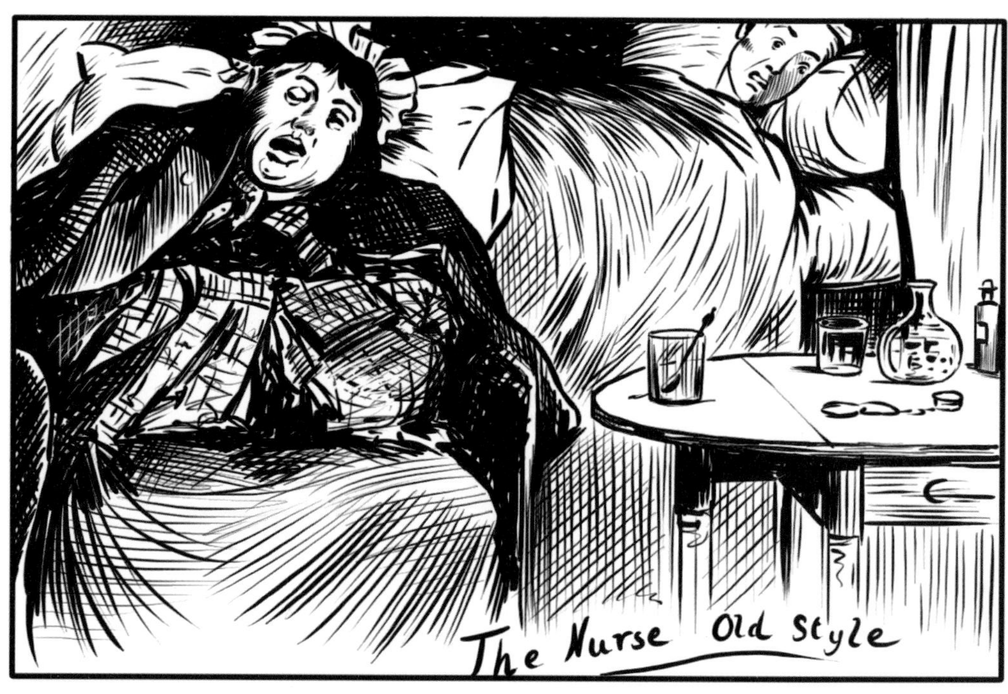

Florence's early career

Florence Nightingale was born in 1820. Her family was wealthy and all they wanted was for her to marry a rich man. They did not expect her to get a job. Florence, however, had different ideas and became interested in nursing.

Secretly, Florence visited hospitals and read about them. She found conditions terrible in most of them. Eventually, she told her parents that she wanted to be a nurse. They were horrified and tried to change her mind.

In 1851, Florence went to Germany to work in a hospital for three months. She returned to London where she got her first job running a hospital for sick 'gentle women'. It was not what she wanted as she wanted to look after the sick.

The Crimean War 1854–56

In 1854, a war broke out between Britain and Russia which was mainly fought in an area known as the Crimea. The army set up hospitals to care for the wounded, but conditions were so bad that almost half the wounded soldiers died. Something had to be done. Florence agreed to lead a team of nurses to the Crimea. She found conditions even worse than expected. There were too few surgeons, no male nurses, and insufficient bandages and beds. The hospital, especially the bed linen, was filthy.

She immediately brought about enormous changes. All the wards were scrubbed clean after the accumulated filth had been removed in wheelbarrows. The windows were opened and fresh air allowed to circulate through the wards. Proper kitchens were set up. Florence reduced the death rate at the hospital from 42% to 2%. The newspapers back in Britain called her 'The Lady with the Lamp'.

 Medicine Through Time

Improvements in nursing

A school for nurses

After her return to England, Florence wrote her ideas on nursing and hospitals in *Notes on Nursing*. She raised £50 000 to set up the Nightingale School of Nursing at St Thomas' Hospital in 1860. This set the pattern for the training of nurses. Every major hospital set up a training school and used her ideas.

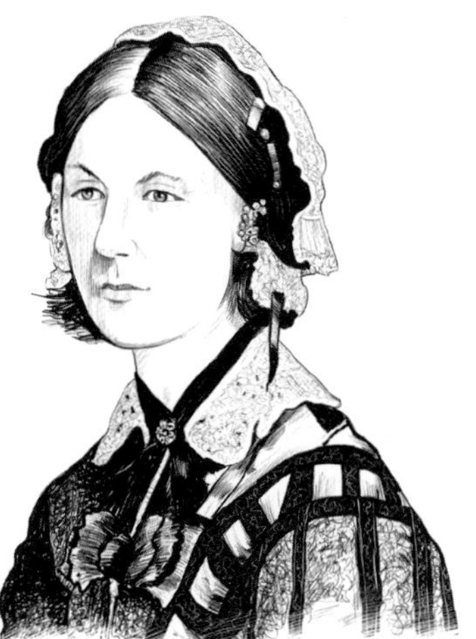

She emphasised a number of points that every nurse should follow.
- Nursing required total dedication.
- Nurses also had to understand medical procedures. This was very important if the nurse was to be able to assist the doctor. All-round medical training was essential.
- They were to keep detailed records of all patients. Florence organised records of admissions, discharges, types of illness, treatment and deaths.

Nursing became much more popular as a career and many girls were attracted. In 1861, there were 24 821 nurses. By 1901, this had nearly trebled to 61 159.

Design of hospitals

Florence also improved the design of hospitals. She believed it very important to have fresh air and sunlight for patients. She also considered it essential to have plenty of space and a design which made for easy cleaning.

Her importance

Florence Nightingale is important for three main reasons.
- She improved the design of hospitals.
- She turned nursing into a popular and trained profession.
- She improved the position of women. In Victorian times, women were expected to stay in the background and let men make all the decisions. Florence refused to do this and showed that women could play an important role in medical improvements.

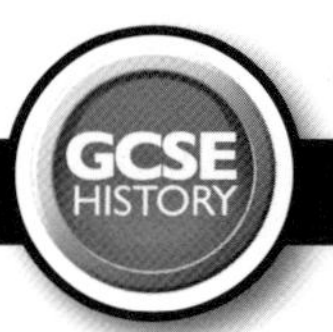

Improvements in hospitals

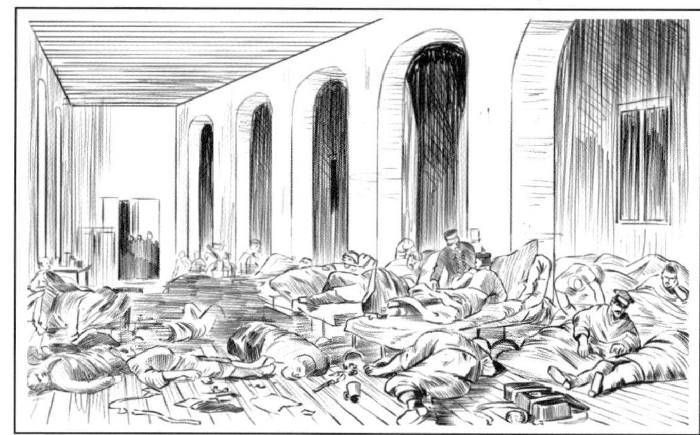

The hospital at Scutari before Florence arrived.

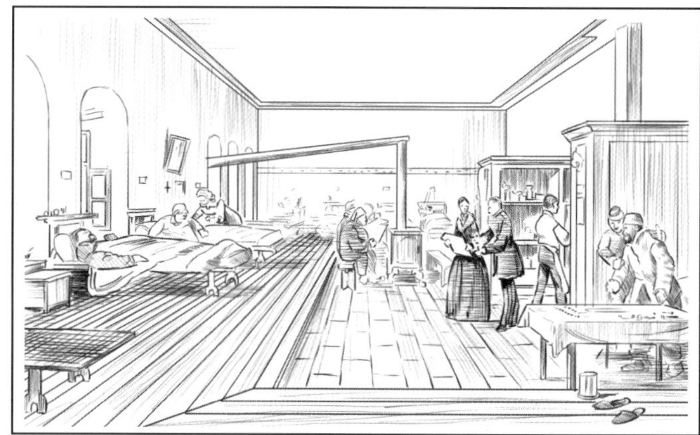

The hospital ward after the changes introduced by Florence.

Write down three improvements in the hospital.

1. ....

2. ....

3. ....

Obituary

When famous people die, newspapers write an obituary of their life. This summarises their main achievements. Write your own obituary on Florence Nightingale. It has been started for you.

Yesterday, Florence Nightingale died. She had many achievements. These included…

....

....

....

....

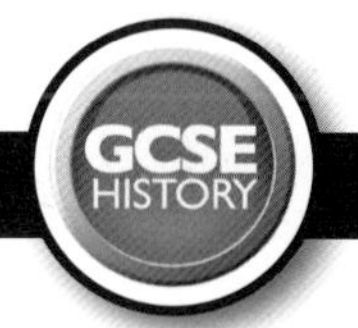

Inferences

You are often asked to make inferences from sources. This means to get 'messages' from the source or to 'read between the lines'. What tone or attitude does the author have? Is he or she angry?

- As you read the source, underline words or phrases that give you a message.
- Messages can be as little as one word, for example, 'the person is *happy*'.
- Begin your answer with 'This source suggests…'

Read Source A. What can you learn from Source A about conditions in the hospital at Scutari?

Source A: A newspaper reporter describes the hospital at Scutari before Florence arrived.

> No sufficient preparations had been made for the care of the wounded. Not only were there insufficient surgeons, not only are there no dressers or male nurses, there is not even enough linen to make bandages.

Here is one inference:
Source A suggests that there was poor organisation at the hospital (shortages of surgeons and bandages).

Here is another inference:
Source A also suggests that many patients will not be treated (shortage of nurses and surgeons).

Now have a go yourself. Read Source B. What can you learn from Source B about the work of Florence Nightingale?

Source B: The same newspaper reporter describes Florence's work at Scutari.

> When all the medical officers have retired for the night and silence and darkness have settled…upon those miles of bed ridden sick, she may be observed alone with a little lamp in her hand making her solitary rounds to comfort the patients.

Source B suggests that ....

....

....

....

Source B also suggests that ....

....

....

....

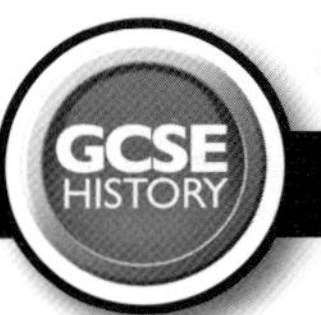

Assessing inferences

Read Source C.

Source C: From a textbook on medicine.

> In six months, Florence Nightingale had cut the death rate of wounded soldiers to only two out of every hundred. The newspapers back home called her 'The Lady with the Lamp'. Supporters raised thousands of pounds.

What can you learn from Source C about Florence Nightingale's work in Scutari?

Here are two answers to the question.

Candidate A

Florence Nightingale was obviously very successful in her work at hospital because she had greatly reduced the death rate. In addition, she had become very popular because of her image as 'The Lady with the Lamp'. People were prepared to help her by donating money.

Candidate B

In six months at Scutari, Florence Nightingale managed to cut the death rate of wounded soldiers to only two out of every hundred. In addition, the newspapers in England called her 'The Lady with the Lamp'. Supporters raised thousands of pounds

Assess each answer.

▸ As you read the answer, underline any inference/message the candidate makes.
▸ Give each answer a level, using the mark scheme below, with a reason for your decision.

Level 1	Summarises or copies out the source.
Level 2	Makes at least one inference from the source.

	Level	Reason
A		
B		

Medicine Through Time

© Folens (copiable page)

(✓) Tick the boxes to show what you know.

I know:

	know / yes	not sure / sometimes	don't know / no
what nursing was like in the early 19th century			
why conditions were so bad at Scutari hospital			
how Florence Nightingale improved conditions in the hospital			
why Florence Nightingale was known as the 'Lady with the Lamp'			
how Florence Nightingale improved nursing when she returned to Britain			
Florence Nightingale's overall importance			
how to compare two illustrations			
how to write an obituary			
what is meant by an inference			
how to make inferences from sources			

I know best:

....

I need to work on (up to three targets):

....

....

....

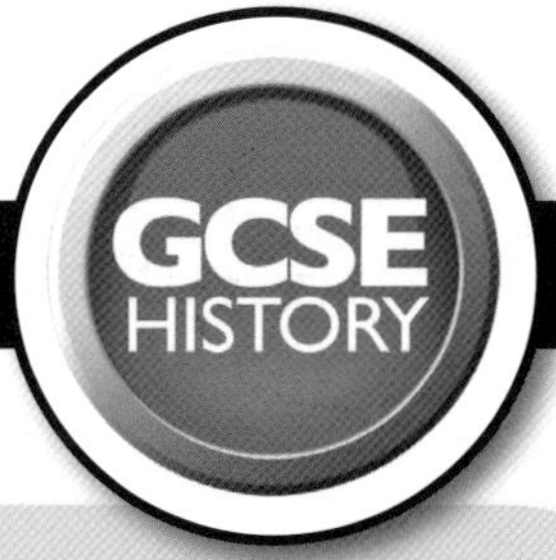

Developments in germ theory and vaccination, 1750–1900

Objectives

▶ Understand the key developments in germ theory and vaccination
▶ Be able to rank order of importance of individuals
▶ Understand how to cross-reference two sources
▶ Be able to assess own progress

Prior knowledge

To achieve these objectives, students should have a reading age of 11–12 years and should have some understanding of source skills. They should also be able to comprehend and interpret written sources.

Links with GCSE specifications

Edexcel: Medicine
AQA: Medicine and Public Health Through Time
OCR: Medicine Through Time

▶ Key study area
▶ Source cross-referencing skills

Background

In the mid to late 19th century, scientists reached an important turning point. They proved that germs caused disease. Pasteur and Koch were able to build on the work of Edward Jenner who, accidentally, discovered a vaccine against smallpox. For centuries, sense had told people that there was a connection between dirt and disease, but they had not been able to explain what the link was. In the early 1800s, the popular explanation was miasma or bad air. Poisonous fumes (called miasma) were given off from rubbish and decaying matter. The fumes were swept from one place to another by the wind.

Starter activity

Carry out a role-play exercise involving two students, Students A and B, to develop cross-referencing skills. Ensure the students have similar and different clothing. Pose the question 'Does Student B support Student A in what they are wearing'? Ask the whole class to cross-reference similarities and differences. Obtain feedback to reinforce cross-referencing skills.

Resource sheets and activity sheets

For resource sheets 'The work of Jenner' and 'The work of Pasteur and Koch', students could work in pairs or groups to research one of the key people and feed back to the whole class. They could be asked to give the importance of the work of each individual a rating of 1–5, with 5 being important and 1 unimportant. This should help students in making their judgements for activity sheet 'Who made the greatest contribution?'. Stress the need for the students to justify their rank order.

For 'Who made the greatest contribution', students should decide whether they think Jenner, Pasteur or Koch made the greatest contribution to medical science between 1750 and 1900.

'Cross-referencing sources' requires the students to read the sources together and highlight any similarities and differences.

On 'Cross-referencing sources: How to answer', students could work in pairs. Ensure they make suggestions as to how the answer could be improved to Level 2.

Plenary

The rivalry between Pasteur and Koch was intensified by their different nationalities – Pasteur was French and Koch was German; France had recently been defeated and humiliated by Germany. Divide the students in half and ask them to produce newspaper headlines on:

▶ praising the work of Pasteur;
▶ criticising the work of Koch.

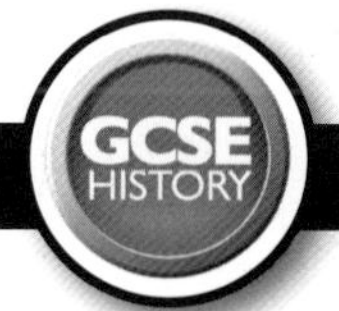

The work of Jenner

Discovery

Edward Jenner worked as a doctor in Gloucestershire. He discovered from local farmers that people believed that they could not catch smallpox if they had already had a mild disease called cowpox. Jenner found this was the case with dairy maids. He decided to use this cowpox as a vaccination.

Use

He tried this with 23 different cases and found that it protected those people against smallpox. He called this technique 'vaccination' after the Latin word for cow 'vacca'. By 1803, doctors were using Jenner's technique in the USA. In 1805, Napoleon had his soldiers vaccinated. In 1852, the British government made vaccination compulsory.

Opposition

As with most new ideas, some people opposed Jenner's methods. Vaccination was seen as dangerous. Some doctors were not as careful as Jenner and their patients died. Others refused to accept the evidence that Jenner had recorded.

His importance

Jenner did not know how his vaccine worked. Nevertheless, his vaccination undoubtedly saved many lives. He was the first immuniser and made deliberate use of the knowledge that recovering from a mild form of a disease gives humans protection (or immunity) from a more serious form. This is the basis of the science of immunology.

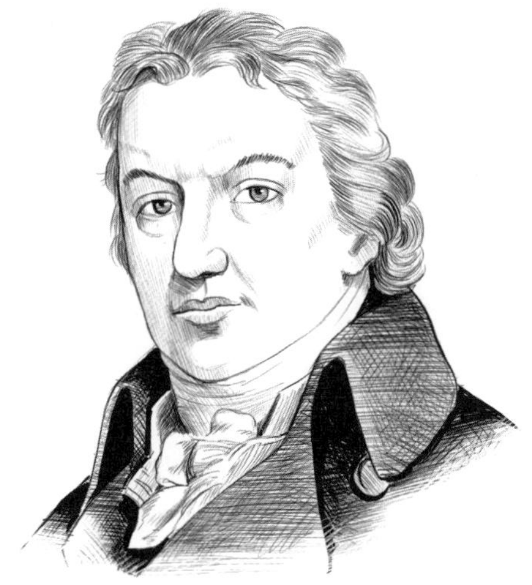

Jenner

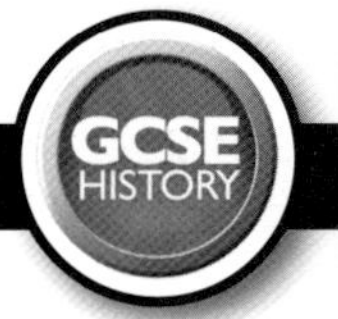

The work of Pasteur and Koch

	Pasteur (1822–95)	**Koch** (1843–1910)
Their work	He was a French chemist who developed a theory that germs multiplied through fermentation. He discovered tiny creatures in various liquids such as wine and milk. By heating up and cooling down the liquid, he was able to get rid of the creatures or germs. This became known as pasteurization.	He was a German physician who came from a poor family. He read up all the latest ideas, especially those of Pasteur. He discovered germs that caused disease by growing the germs in a single glass plate and studying it carefully with a microscope.
Their importance	Pasteur managed to prove that germs come from the air and are not made from the liquids. He did this by heating two lots of liquids, one of which was sealed up and the other of which wasn't. After a few days, he found that the one that was not sealed up had germs but the other had none. Pasteur found that these germs or microbes lived in many things and caused disease. He examined the blood of unhealthy people and found these germs. He found vaccinations for anthrax and chickenpox.	Once he had discovered the cause of a disease, it was possible for other people to find cures for it and to produce vaccines. His methods were copied by other scientists such as Paul Ehrlich who was one of his team. Ehrlich used coloured chemical dyes in the body to show up germs. Koch is therefore associated with the beginning of the science of microbiology. He identified the microbe responsible for tuberculosis.
Failures and limitations	He was able to identify the germ that caused cholera but was unable to find a cure.	He claimed to have found a cure for tuberculosis. This was not very effective.

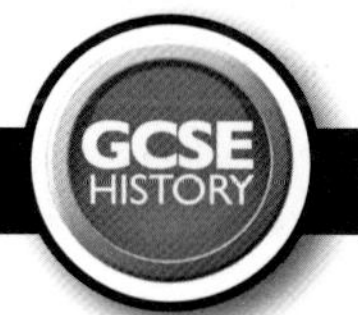

Who made the greatest contribution?

Decide who made the greatest contribution to medical science in the years 1750–1900: Jenner, Pasteur or Koch?

▸ Write the name of the most important in the centre circle and give an explanation of his work and why he was so important.

▸ Write the name of the least important on the outside circle. Explain his work and why it was less important.

▸ Write the name of the third individual in the middle circle, explaining his work and the reason for your choice.

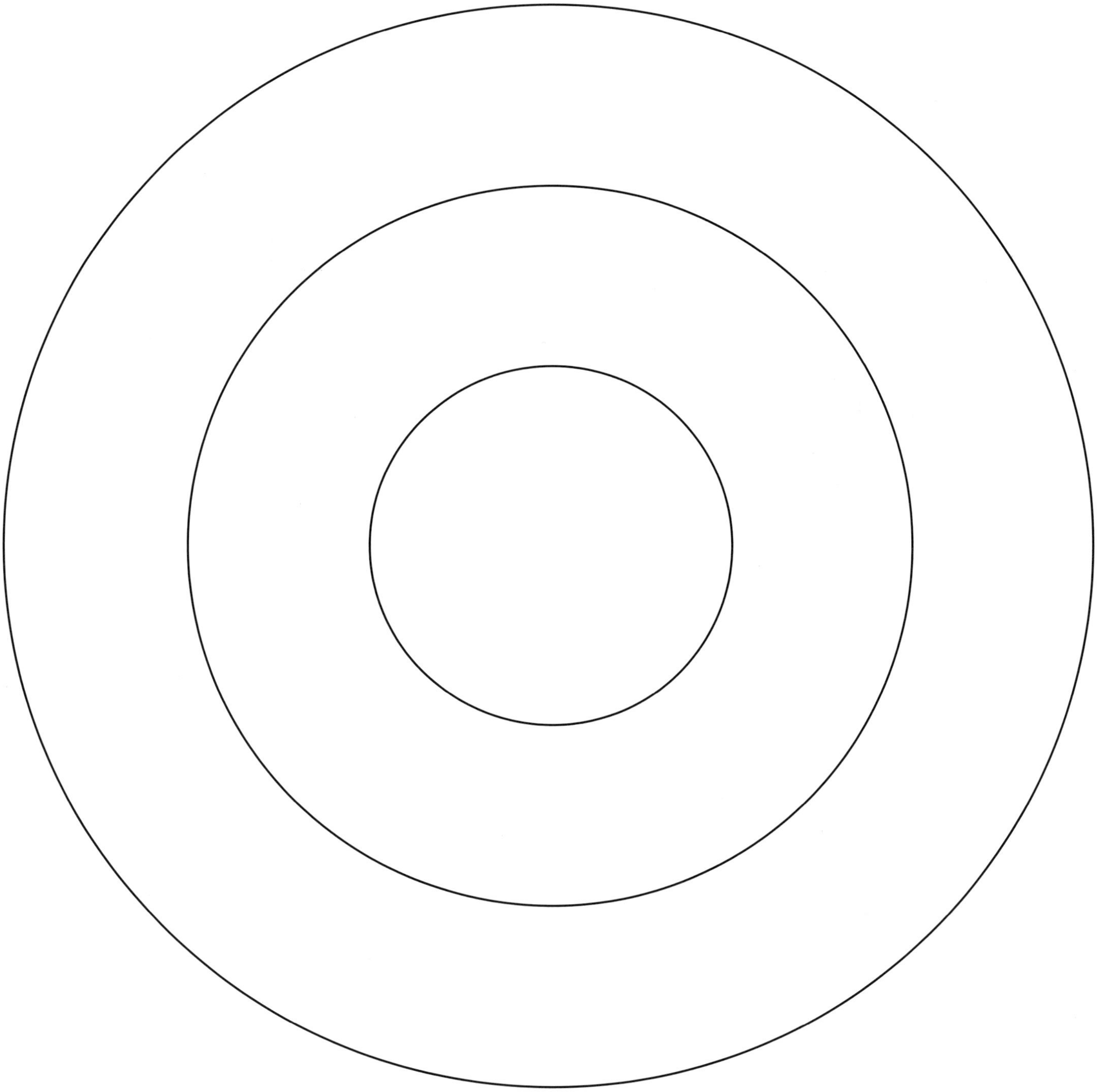

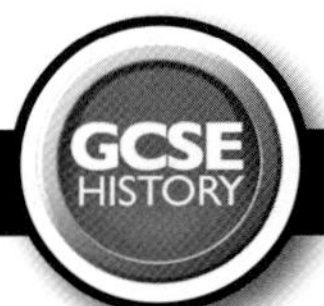

Cross-referencing sources

Source A: From *A History of Medicine* written in 1977.

> Jenner's introduction of vaccination stands as one of the most beneficial changes in the history of medicine. He did not know the cause of disease but his work is recognised as the starting point of attempts to stop infection through immunization.

Source B: From *Disease and its Control* written in 1983.

> In truth, Jenner's work turned out to be a dead end. His discovery was due to a natural fluke of sorts, on the act that a virus that caused a relatively harmless human disease, cowpox, provided immunity against deadly smallpox. He had no understanding of the cause of the disease and made no contribution in this area.

Does Source B support the evidence of Source A about the importance of the work of Jenner? Explain your answer.

▸ Read each source and in one colour highlight any areas of support between the two sources.

▸ In a different colour, highlight any differences.

Now plan your answer using the following grid. One example has been done for you.

	Support	**Differences**
Evidence from Source B		Beneficial change.
Evidence from Source A		Turned out to be a dead end.

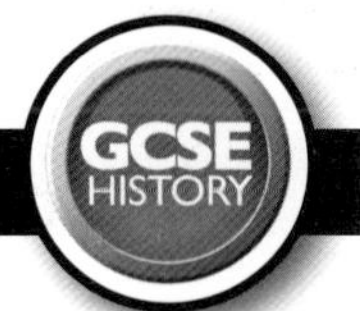

Cross-referencing sources: How to answer

Look at Sources A and B on activity sheet 'Cross-referencing sources'.

Now write your answer using the frame below.

Source B supports Source A because Source B suggests that ....

....

This supports Source A which suggests that ....

....

Source B does not support Source A because Source B suggests that ....

....

....

Whereas Source A suggests that ....

....

....

What level would you give the following answer? Complete the grid and suggest how the answer could be improved.

Level 1	Simple statements about the sources. Students often summarise the contents. Little or no cross-referencing.
Level 2	Developed statements cross-referencing the contents of the two sources.

Candidate's answer

Source A says that Jenner's work is seen as the starting point for immunisation and the fight against disease. Source B says he discovered that cowpox was successful in dealing with smallpox but that this was done through some fluke.

Level	Target to improve

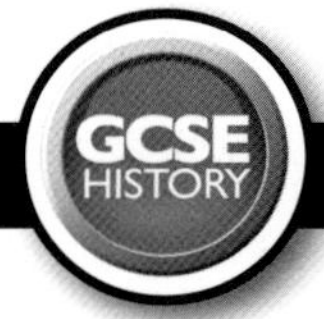

(✓) Tick the boxes to show what you know

I know:

	know / yes	not sure / sometimes	don't know / no
how Jenner discovered a vaccination against smallpox			
why some people at the time opposed his vaccination			
what is meant by pasteurisation			
how Pasteur discovered that germs came from the air			
how Koch encouraged scientific methods			
how to make judgements on the importance of individuals			
how to cross-reference between two sources			
how to achieve Level 2 in cross-referencing			

I know best:

....

I need to work on (up to three targets):

....

....

....

      Medicine Through Time   © Folens (copiable page)

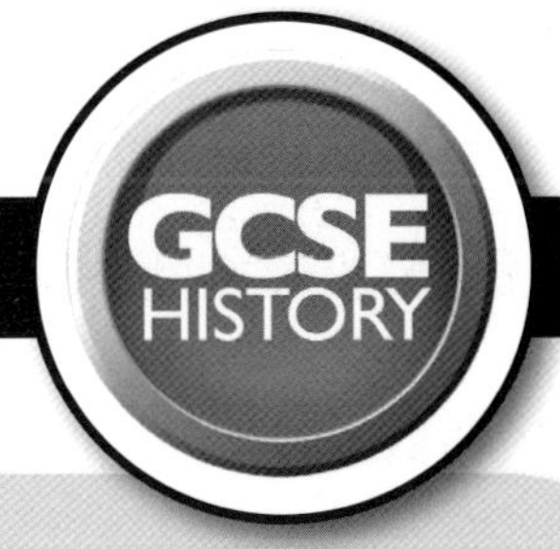

Public health in the 19th century

Objectives

▸ Understand changes in attitudes to public health in the 19th century
▸ Annotate a cartoon
▸ Understand the meaning of interpretations
▸ Be able to assess own progress

Prior knowledge

To achieve these objectives, students should have a reading age of 11–12 years and should have some understanding of source skills. They should also be able to comprehend and interpret written sources.

Links with GCSE specifications

Edexcel: Medicine
AQA: Medicine and Public Health Through Time
OCR: Medicine Through Time

▸ Key study area
▸ Explaining the accuracy of an interpretation

Background

For hundreds of years, people had known that there was a link between dirt and disease. However, no one knew what the connection was. Britain experienced an industrial revolution in the 18th and 19th centuries. This led to the rapid growth of industrial towns which could not cope with the need to house people and provide them with water and facilities to remove their sewage. Towns became overcrowded with little or no sanitation or refuse disposal and infected water supplies. In these conditions, killer diseases, especially cholera, spread easily and quickly. Government and local authorities were reluctant to intervene because of prevailing laissez-faire attitudes and the potential cost.

Starter activity

Discuss the meaning of interpretations. Stress that there is always more than one interpretation of any event or person. Ask the students to write their own interpretation (with reasons) of a TV soap. Volunteers should read out their interpretations. Ask the students to decide on the accuracy of these interpretations. How did they decide?

Resource sheets and activity sheets

For 'Cholera', put the class in groups and pose the question 'Were the newspaper headlines justified?' Give each group one headline and ask them to write an imaginary report on cholera. Obtain whole class feedback.

Encourage individual research on 'Improvements in public health'. Students could be asked to decide which was the most important change brought in by the government and why.

Provide a careful briefing for activity sheet 'Public health reasons for the spread of disease' and encourage volunteers to read out their annotations and suggestions to reduce the possibility of disease.

For 'Interpretations of the cholera epidemics', students could work in pairs to match the inferences to the interpretations. The first one could be done as a whole class activity. (Answers: 1. Source D; 2. Source A; 3. Source C; 4. Source B; 5. Source F; 6. Source E.)

'Accuracy of interpretations' could, initially, be done as a whole class exercise when deciding what is accurate about the interpretation.

Plenary

Ask two students to imagine they are in a lift. The lift takes one minute to go from floors 1 to 10. During the journey up, one student has to tell the other all they know about cholera in the 19th century. On the way down, the other student tells all they know about government and local authority improvements in public health in the 19th century.

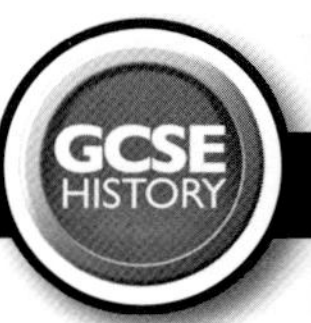

Cholera

No rank escapes its attack

Whole families exterminated

CIVILIZED NATIONS REDUCED TO SAVAGE HORDES!

Cholera was a new disease to Britain. In fact, it was unknown before 1831 but was thought to have come from India. Cholera struck for the first time in 1831 and returned in 1848, 1853 and 1866. It was frightening because it was a 'shock disease' that struck quickly. Sufferers were suddenly gripped by diarrhoea and vomiting. It was a swift, painful and unpleasant death.

Causes

What people believed at the time	Its actual causes
Contagionists believed that cholera was spread by personal contact – via the person or clothes or bedding. Miasmatists were convinced that cholera was carried through the air, something like an infectious mist. Ignorance of its causes made it difficult to stop the spread of the disease. Indeed, one suggested cure was imported Japanese cheroots as their fragrance was supposed to remove cholera.	Cholera is actually spread by infected water. The faeces of a sufferer will contain the cholera germ and if these germs get into the water supply, the disease spreads rapidly. In 1854, Dr John Snow showed there was a link between cholera and water from the Thames. He proved that 500 cases of cholera were linked to a water pump in the Broad Street area of London. Louis Pasteur proved the existence of cholera bacteria and Koch established the precise cause.

Other problems

Cholera was the most frightening disease but it was far from the only danger to health. Bad water supplies, inadequate drains, damp houses and rubbish lining the streets all helped spread disease. These brought diarrhoea, typhoid and cholera. Governments and public authorities were reluctant to intervene to try to improve public health.

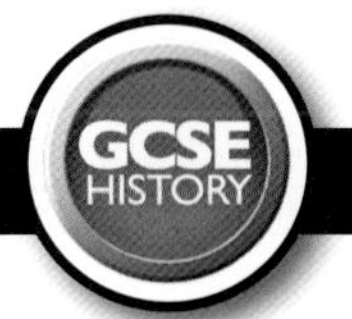

Improvements in public health

Edwin Chadwick

He was a government official who supervised the help that was given to the poor. He wrote a report on the living conditions and health of the poor in the towns in 1842. His report suggested that much poverty was due to ill health which, in turn, was due to the foul conditions in which people lived. He suggested that local authorities should improve public health.

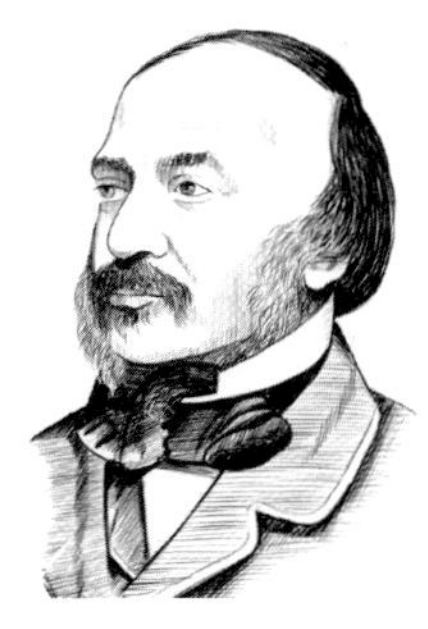

Chadwick

There was much opposition to Chadwick's report and the idea of government and local authority help.

- Many believed in 'laissez-faire' or leave to do – the idea that governments should interfere as little as possible.
- Improvements in public health would cost money. This would lead to an increase in local rates. Local businessmen wanted to keep the rates down.

Why did government become involved?

This was due to:
- further cholera epidemics in the 1850s and 1860s;
- reports such as that of Chadwick, 1842, and Dr Southwood-Smith, whose Report on the Health of Towns in 1848 showed again the connection between squalor and overcrowding and the spread of disease.

Date	Change	What it did
1848	Public Health Act	Set up local Boards of Health and Medical Officers, although these were not compulsory. A General Board of Health was established.
1858	Public Health Act	Local Boards of Health were set up but were not controlled by the General Board.
1866	Sanitary Act	Each town was forced to appoint Sanitary Inspectors to end the worst cases of overcrowding.
1872	Public Health Act	Sanitary Authorities were set up and Medical Officers of Health became compulsory.
1875	Public Health Act	Local authorities were given powers to provide water and sanitation. Towns were forced to appoint Health Inspectors.

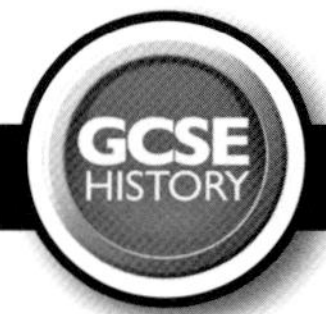

Public health reasons for the spread of disease

Using arrows and annotation, indicate what in this street would have encouraged the spread of disease.

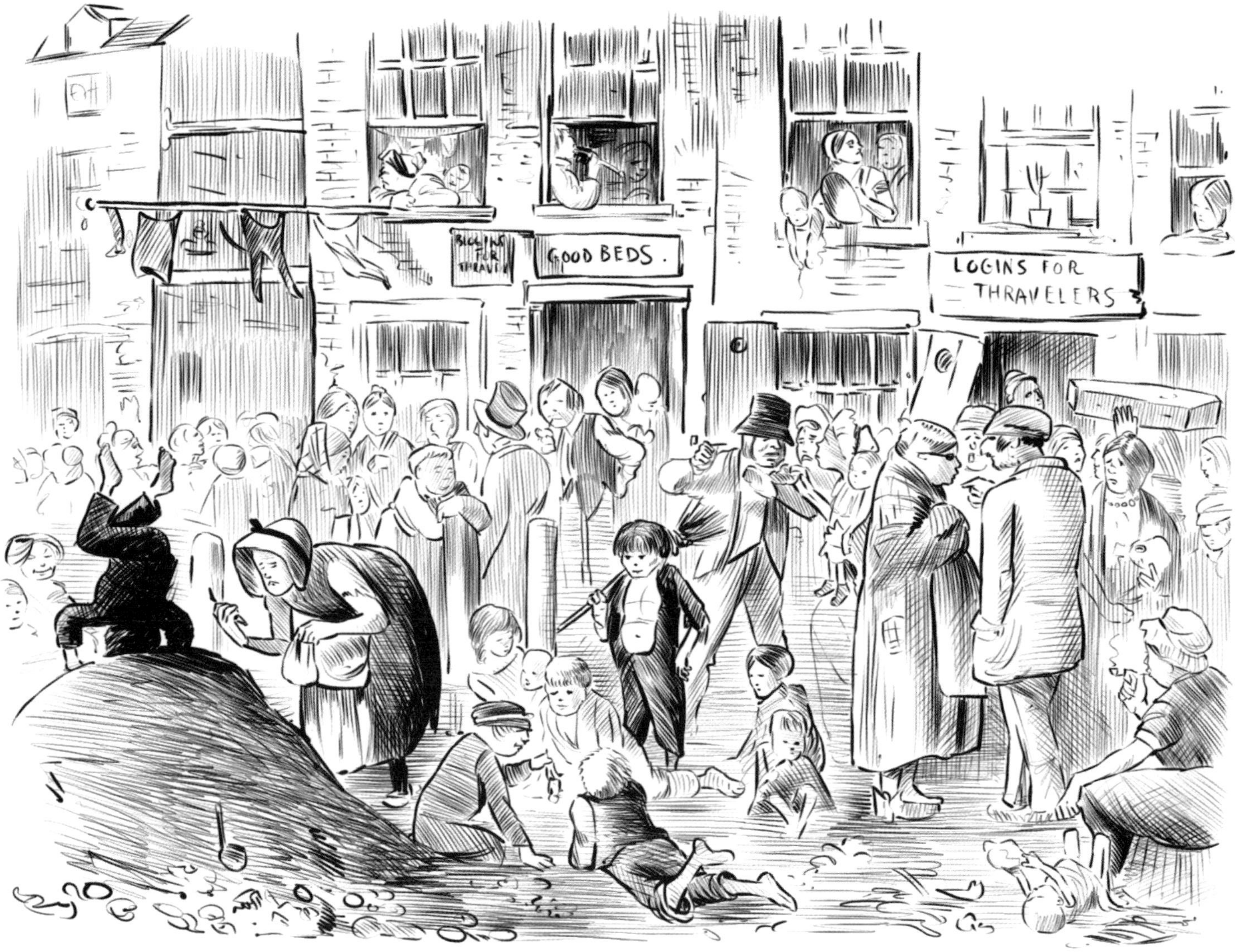

Give two suggestions to improve the health of the residents of this street.

1. ....

....

....

2. ....

....

....

     Medicine Through Time   © Folens (copiable page)

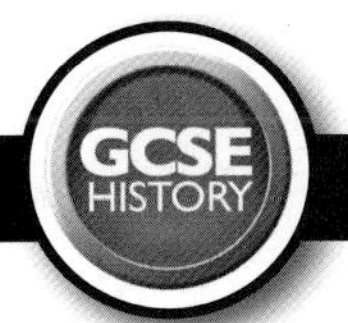

Interpretations of the cholera epidemics

Source A: Edinburgh Board of Health, 1833.

> Experience proves that notorious drunkards are amongst the victims. Also the old, the ill, the poor and prostitutes.

Source B: Bishop Bloomfield, 1832.

> Cholera is a sign to increase the comforts and improve the moral character of the masses.

Source C: Dr Southwood-Smith, 1841.

> Cholera was due not to want of food and great misery but to bad air that carried disease.

Source D: Textbook on medicine, 1996.

> Cholera is actually spread by infected water. The faeces of the sufferer contain a cholera germ and if it gets into the water supply the disease spreads rapidly.

Source E: Thomas Wakely, a doctor, 1831.

> We can only suppose the existence of a poison which moves independently of the wind, of the soil, of all conditions of the air, and of the sea. One that makes mankind the chief agent of its movement.

Source F: Textbook on medicine, 1995.

> Cholera is believed to have come from central India. From there it spread to China, then across the trade routes to Europe. It struck from time to time in the form of epidemics.

Match the interpretations of the sources to the inferences below. Indicate with a tick or a cross whether the interpretation is correct.

Inference	Interpretation	Tick/cross
1. It was passed through human waste.		
2. It was a punishment to people who drank alcohol.		
3. It was carried by something in the air.		
4. It was to warn people to behave better.		
5. It was an epidemic from Asia.		
6. It was some mysterious poison in the air.		

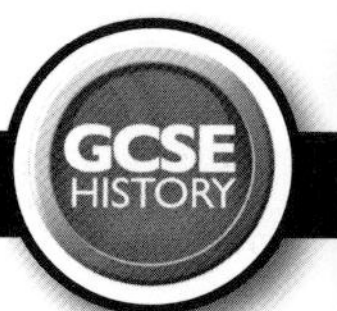

Accuracy of interpretations

You are often asked to judge the accuracy of an interpretation. This means you have to check the accuracy of what the source suggests against your knowledge of the event or person.

Source G: From Edwin Chadwick's *Report on the Sanitary Conditions of the Labouring Population,* **1842.**

> First – That the various forms of epidemic disease among the labouring classes is caused by impurities in the air produced by decaying animal and vegetable substances. These are made worse by filth, bad ventilation and infected water supplies.

Is Source G an accurate view of the reasons for the cholera epidemics of the 19th century?

I believe this is an accurate view because (use your own knowledge to explain the findings of Dr Snow and water):

....

....

....

....

However, I believe this is not fully accurate because Chadwick has the wrong reason for the epidemic. He believes it is caused by (clue: miasma theory):

....

....

....

It is also not accurate because (clue: real cause of cholera):

....

....

....

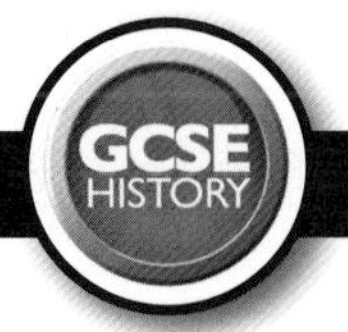

(✓) Tick the boxes to show what you know.

I know:

	know / yes	not sure / sometimes	don't know / no
why cholera was so frightening			
what caused cholera			
what people at the time believed caused cholera			
the importance of Chadwick and Southwood-Smith			
why many people did not want the government involved in public health			
some improvements in public health			
what is meant by an interpretation			
how to decide on the accuracy of an interpretation			

I know best:

....

I need to work on (up to three targets):

....

....

....

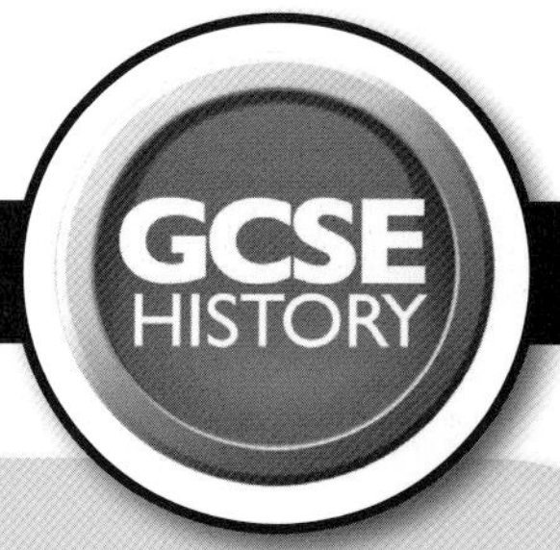

The treatment of disease in the 20th century

Objectives

▸ Understand the developments in the treatment of disease in the 20th century
▸ Understand how to use sources to stimulate own knowledge
▸ Be able to assess own progress

Prior knowledge

To achieve these objectives, students should have a reading age of 11–12 years and should have some understanding of source skills. They should also be able to comprehend and interpret written sources.

Links with GCSE specifications

Edexcel: Medicine
AQA: Medicine and Public Health Through Time
OCR: Medicine Through Time

▸ Key study area
▸ Using sources and own knowledge

Background

Despite the many medical advances of the 19th century, doctors and surgeons were often unable to cure their patients. There were no antibiotics to fight internal infection. Research, led by Pasteur and Koch, was being carried out, in the late 19th century, on all kinds of bacteria. Meanwhile, and separate from this, Charles Darwin developed the theory that various species had evolved through struggle and the 'survival of the fittest'. Some medical scientists saw possibilities here – might not some microbes fight and overcome others? Paul Vuillemin called this process antibiosis. This is the origin of the word antibiotics. Others, such as Ehrlich and Domagk, searched for this antibiotic or 'magic bullet'. The most important development was penicillin, but who really discovered it – was it Fleming or Florey and Chain?

Starter activity

Ask the students what personal examples they can give of treatment for prevention or cure of disease. Prompt them by asking them when they were inoculated, and what against. Have they been prescribed antibiotics for illnesses? Can they remember their names?

Resource sheets and activity sheets

For resource sheets 'The 'magic bullets'' and 'The discovery of penicillin', divide the class into groups. Each group should research 'magic bullets' and penicillin and feed back on how one of the following factors led to their discovery and development – good luck, chance, key individuals, outside (government) help and building on the work of previous research teams or individuals. Hold a class discussion on the most important factors.

Further explain how to use sources to stimulate own knowledge. Students should complete the grid on activity sheet 'Using a source and your own knowledge (1)'. Ask volunteers to read out how they have developed their own knowledge of the highlighted events. Students will need careful guidance as to how to use the sources to stimulate own knowledge for activity sheet 'Using a source and your own knowledge (2)'.

Plenary

Students should be asked to pick one word or phrase relating to key developments under Ehrlich, Domagk and Fleming. Volunteers could carry out a charade/mime illustrating the word, which the rest of the class has to guess. Time how long it takes for the word/phrase to be guessed. This could be followed by a class discussion – who really did discover penicillin?

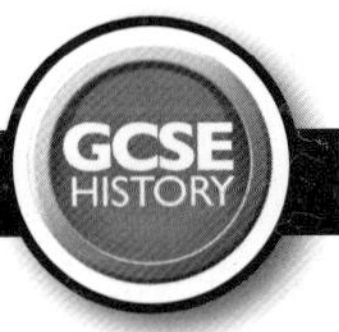

The 'magic bullets'

During the 19th and 20th centuries, doctors and scientists discovered the causes of many illnesses and infectious diseases. However, how could these be cured?

The first magic bullet – Salvarsan 606	The second magic bullet – Protonsil

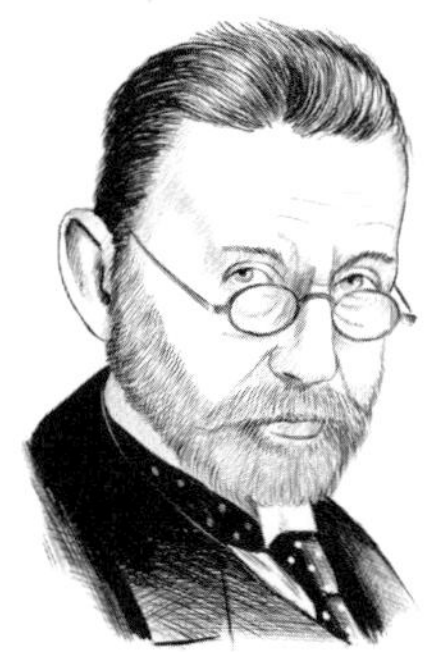

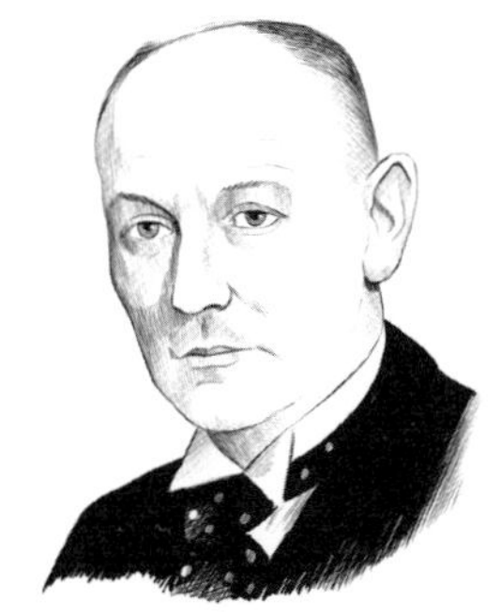

Paul Ehrlich was part of Robert Koch's research team. He followed Koch's ideas of staining bacteria and observing the effects of the dye. He was fascinated by the way the body created antibodies against diphtheria. These antibodies killed the bacteria but did not harm anything else. He called these antibodies 'magic bullets' and was convinced that a chemical could be found that would do the same.

His team tried to find a 'magic bullet' for treating syphilis. They had tried 605 variations when, in 1905, number 606 worked. They nearly missed the discovery of 606, as it was only when it was being re-tested that an assistant, Sahashiro Hata, realised that it killed the syphilis bacteria. This only worked on syphilis.

Ehrlich inspired other researchers to try to find a drug which could be taken internally to destroy harmful bacteria of all kinds.

Research on a second 'magic bullet' was interrupted by the First World War, but in the 1920s it picked up again.

In 1932, Gerhardt Domagk tried out Protonsil, a red dye. He started a series of tests using mice. The results were good. It definitely had an effect on the bacteria that caused blood poisoning.

Much sooner than expected, Domagk tested the drug on a human. His daughter, Hildegarde, was playing with her pet guinea pig near to some medical equipment. She pricked her finger on an infected needle and soon developed severe blood poisoning. With his daughter near to death, Domagk decided to use Protonsil even though it had not been tried on a human being before. He gave her a large dose and she recovered. He had discovered the second 'magic bullet'.

Within two years, French researchers had discovered the key ingredient of Protonsil – sulphonamide, which is derived from coal tar.

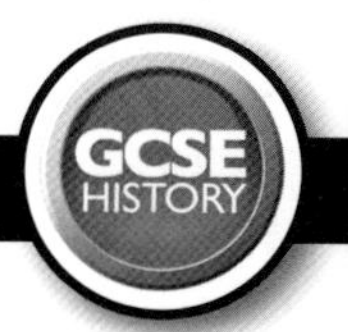

The discovery of penicillin

1928	**1929**	**1937**
Working in his laboratory, Alexander Fleming found that fungus had grown on a dish while he was on holiday. This was by chance, possibly the fungus blew in through an open window. He identified the mould as penicillin.	Fleming published his results, insisting that penicillin could be applied to an infected area and kill the germs. However, he was unable to develop any more penicillin. 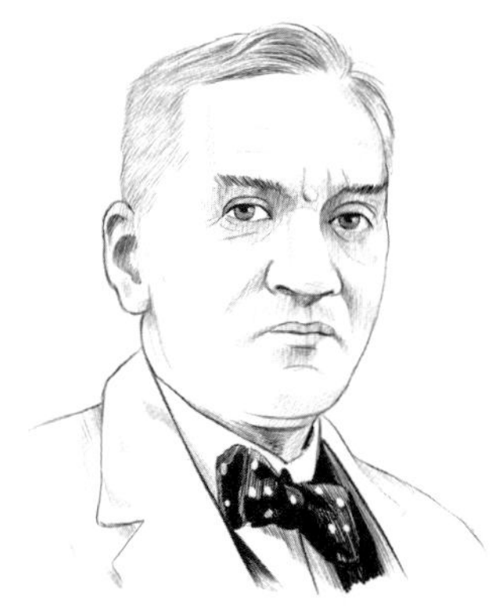	Two Oxford scientists, Howard Florey and Ernst Chain, began to research penicillin after reading an article by Fleming. 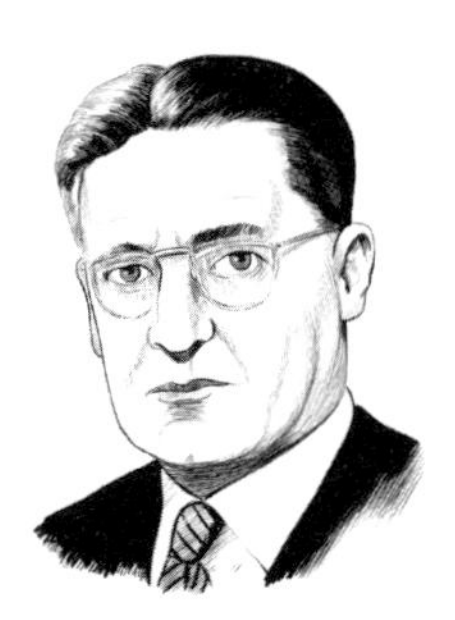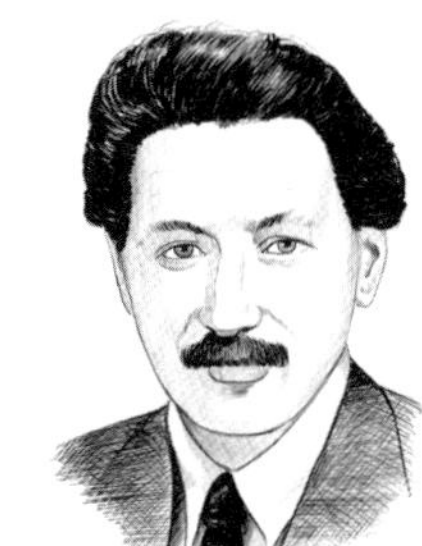
1939	**1940**	**1941**
The two scientists gathered together a skilled research team. The outbreak of the Second World War encouraged the British government to give them research funds. Slowly the team gathered a few grams of pure penicillin.	They experimented on eight mice. All were given dangerous microbes. The four treated with penicillin survived. The other four died.	By 1941, they had enough penicillin to try it on a human being. They tried it on a patient with abscesses all over his face. At first it removed them. However, they ran out of penicillin and the patient died.
1942	**1942**	**1944–45**
Fleming used penicillin on a friend who had meningitis. It was a success.	Florey persuaded the US government to fund the production of penicillin. They agreed to give $80 million to four drug companies to find a way to mass produce it.	By June 1944, there was enough penicillin to treat all the casualties who suffered on D-Day. By 1945, the US army was using two million doses a month.

 Medicine Through Time

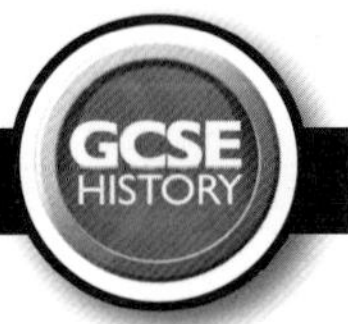

Using a source and own knowledge (I)

You are often asked questions in which you have to use both a source and your own knowledge.

Source A: The discovery of penicillin, written in 1983.

Fleming's role in the discovery of penicillin has generally been exaggerated. He was unable to produce purified penicillin. Credit for purifying penicillin and for overcoming the many problems of mass production belongs to **Howard Florey** and his team of Oxford investigators, most notably **Ernst Chain**, who pointed the group towards penicillin in the first place. Both were helped by the **US government** who paid for the mass production.

Use Source A and your own knowledge to describe the development of penicillin.

The question is asking you to use two things in your answer. Which is more difficult? The best way to do this is to use the source to stimulate your own knowledge. Highlight words, names and dates that you can explain further. For example, certain words have been highlighted in the source.

- Explain what you know about these in the grid below.
- Is there anything else you can expand on? Include in the two blank rows.

Fleming	
Florey and Chain	
US government	

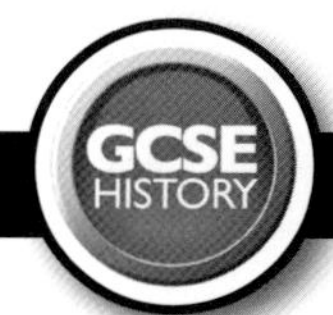

Using a source and own knowledge (2)

Source B: From a modern textbook on medicine.

Ehrlich developed the first magic bullet, known as Salvarson 606. In 1905, his research team tried 605 variations to try to find a cure for syphilis. They nearly missed variation 606 until one of his assistants realised it killed the syphilis bacteria. In 1931, Domagk discovered the second magic bullet, known as Protonsil. It worked on mice and then he used it, far sooner than anticipated, on a human being.

Use Source B and your own knowledge to describe the development of the 'magic bullet'.

Remember to highlight key words, dates or people in the source.

Here is a writing frame to help you.

Using the source

Are there any 'magic bullets' that are well explained in the source and which you can use in your answer?

The source describes the first magic bullet which was ....

....

....

....

....

Using your own knowledge

There is one more 'magic bullet' described. Use your own knowledge to describe its development.

From my own knowledge ....

....

....

....

....

     Medicine Through Time   © Folens (copiable page)

Assessment sheet – The treatment of disease in the 20th century

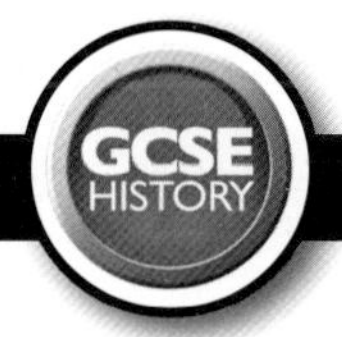

(✓) Tick the boxes to show what you know.

I know:

	know / yes	not sure / sometimes	don't know / no
what is meant by 'magic bullet'			
why the work of Ehrlich was important			
how Domagk tested Protonsil on a human much sooner than expected			
how Fleming accidentally discovered penicillin			
the importance of the work of Florey and Chain			
how the USA helped the mass production of penicillin			
how to use a source to stimulate my own knowledge			
how to write an answer using a source and my own knowledge			

I know best:

....

I need to work on (up to three targets):

....

....

....

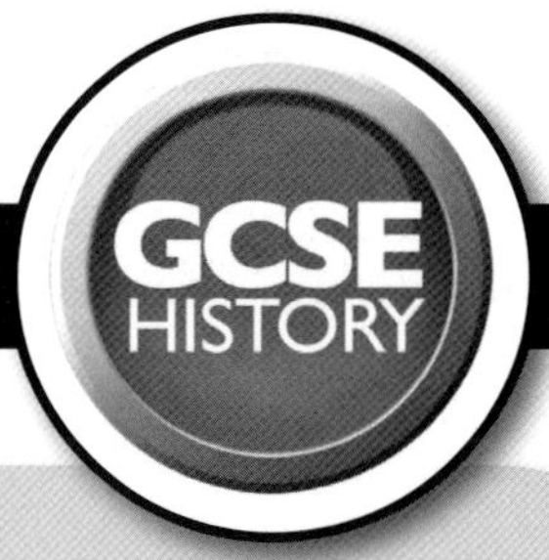

The introduction of the National Health Service

Objectives

- Understand the reasons for and achievements of the NHS
- Organise events chronologically
- Understand how to explain the utility of a source
- Be able to assess own progress

Prior knowledge

To achieve these objectives, students should have a reading age of 11–12 years and should have some understanding of source skills. They should also be able to comprehend and interpret written sources.

Links with GCSE specifications

Edexcel: Medicine
AQA: Medicine and Public Health Through Time
OCR: Medicine Through Time

- Key study area
- Utility of a source

Background

The NHS was the culmination of a series of reforms in the first half of the 20th century which increased the role of government and provided the foundations for the welfare state. The Liberal governments of 1905–14 established the principle of national insurance for both health and unemployment. The Depression of the 1930s highlighted the plight of the unemployed who, in a series of surveys, were shown to be unable to provide for the needs of their families. Life expectancy, diet and health were all shown to be worse in the 'depressed areas'. The final impetus came from the Second World War, during which government intervention, especially rationing, was shown to have real benefits for the whole population. In addition, the war encouraged the idea of creating a better world. The Beveridge Report of 1942 strongly recommended a comprehensive system of national insurance and a national health service. The Labour Party won the general election of 1945 and Aneurin Bevan introduced the NHS Bill in 1946. He faced powerful opposition from the majority of doctors who did not want to be civil servants and so he had to compromise and agree to some private patients. On 5th July 1948, the NHS began.

Starter activity

Students should work in pairs. Using a mind map, with NHS as the central box, they should think of as many services provided by the NHS as they can. They could be helped by clues of key words such as hospitals, dentists, doctors and so on. Obtain feedback and build up a whole class mind map.

Resource sheets and activity sheets

Resource sheet 'Why was the NHS introduced?' and activity sheet 'The road to the NHS' should be used simultaneously. The completed 'The road to the NHS' could be used to prompt discussion about the reasons for the NHS. Students could be asked to prioritise these and give a reason for their choices.

'Achievements of the NHS' could be done as a paired activity. One student researches the benefits and the other the shortcomings. Each teaches the other what they have researched.

For 'Source utility', students could be encouraged to highlight useful content and the provenance of the source. Obtain feedback from the students on the different levels and encourage them to give reasons for their decisions.

Explain the planning grid for 'Writing an answer'. Encourage students, in their planning, to use the Level 2 answers. Stress the importance of using the words 'useful' and 'limitations' in their answers.

Plenary

Put students into groups. Each group should consider and give feedback on the following:

- Do the benefits outweigh the shortcomings of the NHS?
- Should the NHS or private practice be abolished?
- Provide one suggestion to improve the NHS.

Obtain feedback and carry out a class discussion.

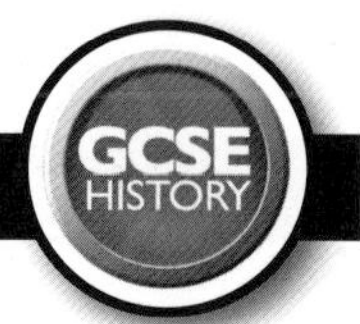

Why was the NHS introduced?

In 1948, the National Health Service was introduced in Britain. This was due to several reasons.

5 July 1948

The first day of the NHS. Hospitals were taken over by the government. Free medical and dental treatment. A fairer distribution of doctors throughout the country.

National Insurance Act

This was introduced in 1911. Workers and their employers made weekly contributions to a central fund which was then used to give workers sickness benefit and free medical treatment. This did not include their families.

NHS Bill

In 1946, the NHS Bill was introduced by Aneurin Bevan.

The Second World War, 1939–45

This forced the government to do much more to improve the health of the people. Rationing ensured that everyone had a reasonable diet and the health of the people improved.

New Labour Government 1945

In 1945, the Labour Party won the general election. Its members were committed to the idea of a National Health Service.

The Depression of the 1930s

Britain suffered from high unemployment in the 1930s. The worst-hit areas were known as the 'depressed areas'. Several surveys were done which showed that the health, living conditions and diet of these people was far worse than those in areas of employment. There were calls for a NHS.

The Beveridge Report 1942

Beveridge wrote a famous report in which he suggested a free national health service as part of a new scheme of national insurance. He talked about looking after people from the 'cradle to the grave'.

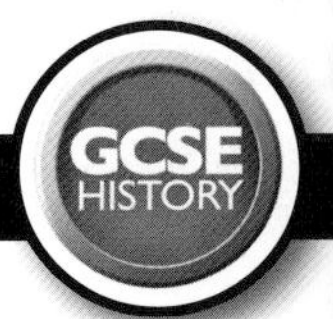

Achievements of the NHS

Achievements	Shortcomings
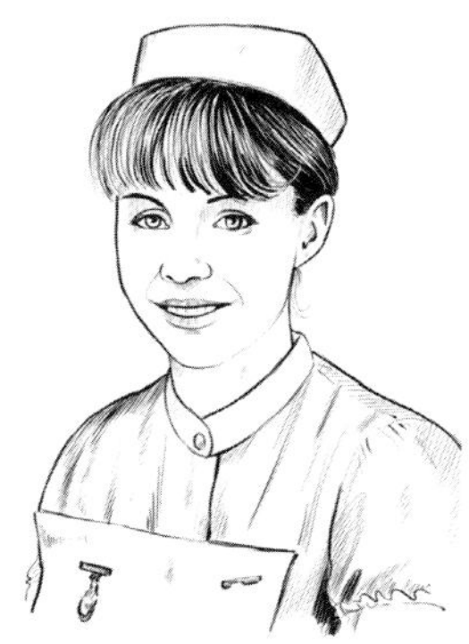	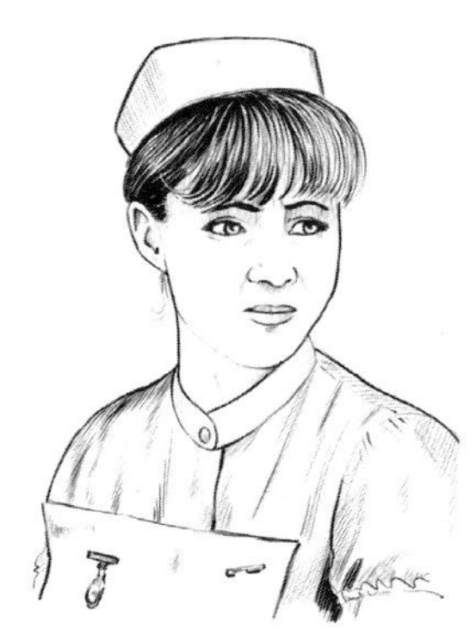

Achievements

Medical treatment was now available to rich and poor alike.

The first few days of the NHS were astonishing. A flood of patients sought treatment after a lifetime of suffering. By 1951, the NHS had given out 187 million prescriptions and 5.25 million pairs of glasses and dentists had treated 8.5 million patients.

It took away the worry about money in time of sickness.

The NHS made women's health a priority. Women are now four times more likely to consult a doctor than a man. Life expectancy for women has risen from 66 to 78. Maternal mortality has been reduced.

The NHS costs less than other systems. For example, the USA has a private health care system which costs 12% of national income while the NHS costs 6%.

It has transformed the role of the family doctor. GPs increasingly work as part of teams offering a whole range of health services.

Shortcomings

Many doctors were against the NHS because they did not want to be employed by the government and be told where to work. Bevan won most over by promising they would be allowed private patients.

Others have criticised private health treatment which often seems to be quicker and better than the NHS.

The cost of the NHS soared in the years after 1948. Indeed, in its first year it cost £400 million. The government therefore brought in charges for prescriptions and dental treatment.

It has encouraged many people, some not genuinely ill, to visit their doctors or local hospital.

Others believe it has encouraged many people to be too dependent on the state. This has been described as a 'nanny state'.

In recent years, lack of money in the NHS has left hospital beds unused even though there is a need for them.

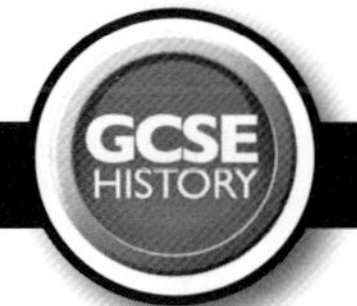

The road to the NHS

The reasons for the NHS are in the wrong order. Put them in the right sequence. Write the reasons on the 'road to the NHS' below.

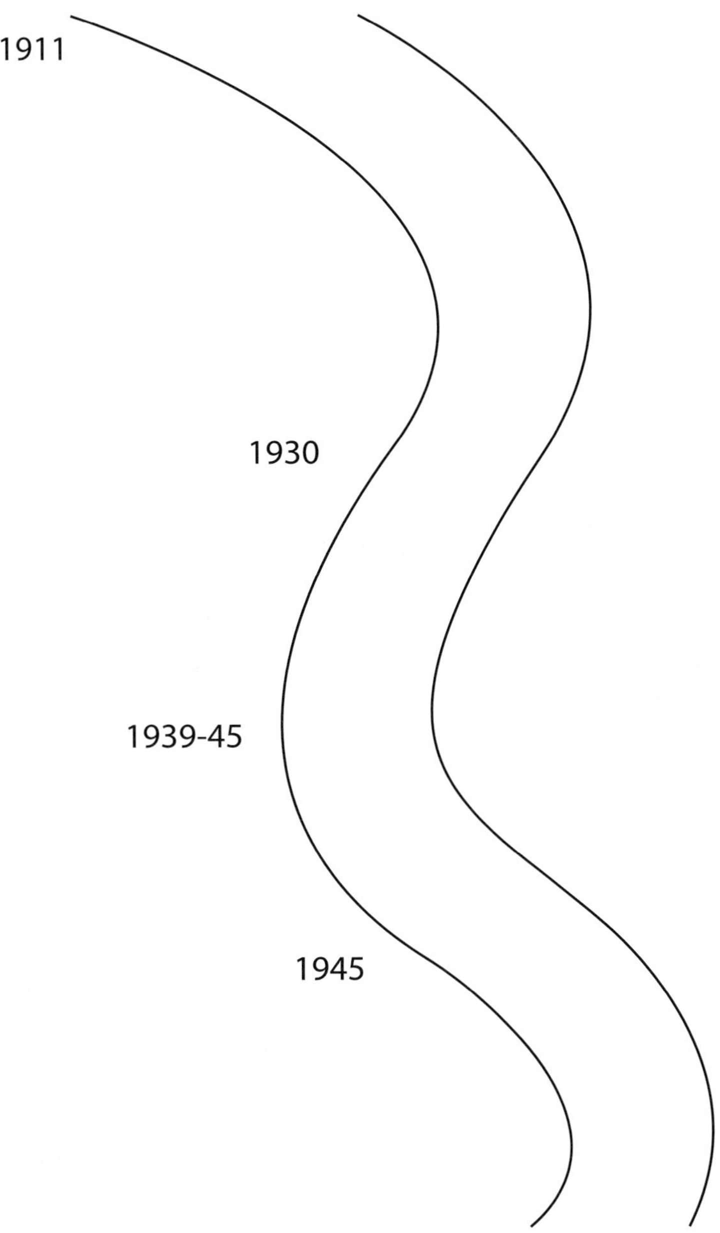

The following is from a student who has revised the NHS. However, he has not revised thoroughly and has made several mistakes. Re-write the account and correct his mistakes.

The National Health Service was introduced in 1958 by Beveridge, the Labour minister. This was partly due to the Bevan Report of 1933 which recommended looking after people from the grave to the cradle. Doctors fully supported its introduction. The NHS cost £200 million in its first year.

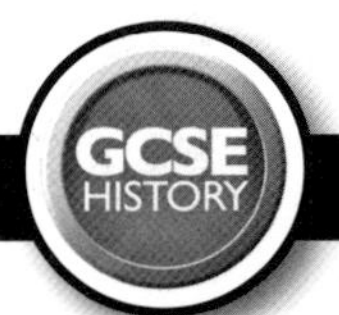

Source utility

You are often asked to explain the utility of a source. This means how useful the source is.

Source A: Alice Law, recalling, in the 1960s, the first day of the NHS, 5 July 1948.

> My mother went and got tested for new glasses. Then she went further down the road for the chiropodist. She had her feet done. Then she went back to the doctor's because she'd been having trouble with her ears and the doctor said he would fix her up with a hearing aid. I remember her saying to the doctor on the way out, 'Well, the undertaker's on the way home, I might as well call in there'.

How useful is Source A as evidence of the changes brought about by the NHS?

Level 1	Generalised statements that could apply to any source, for example, 'It is no good because it exaggerates'. Summarises the contents of the source. No mention of utility.
Level 2	Developed statements which focus on the utility of the contents and/or the provenance of the source.

Here is a set of statements. Which are Level 1 and which are Level 2?

Statement	Level
This source is no good because it was written later.	
This source is useful because it was written by someone whose mother experienced the start of the NHS.	
This source is useful because it suggests that people got immediate benefits from the NHS such as hearing aids and spectacles.	
This source is no good because it is biased.	
Source A says that her mother went and got tested for new glasses and then went to the chiropodist.	
The source is of limited use because it is one-sided. It only gives the view of someone who benefited from the NHS.	
Source A is of limited use because it does not explain the experiences of other patients for the NHS.	
The source is useful because it suggests that the NHS brought great benefits to many patients who, at last, could get much needed treatment.	
The source says that the mother decided to call in to the undertaker's on the way home.	

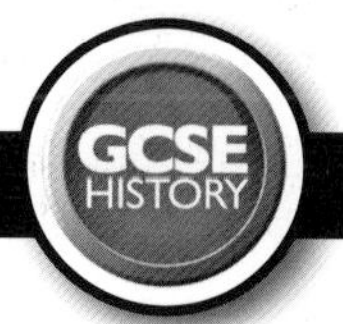

Writing an answer

First plan your answer in the grid below. Use the Level 2 statements from 'Source utility'.

Contents What is useful about what the source is suggesting?	Source A is useful because it suggests…
Provenance This is the information given above the source. It may be useful because of the date it was produced and who produced it.	It is also useful because…
Limitations This means it is less useful because it only gives one side. Whose side? It gives a limited view – what is not shown or explained?	It has limitations because…

Write your answers below.

Source A is useful because it suggests ....

....

....

It is also useful because it suggests that ....

....

It is useful because it was (provenance of source) ....

....

It is of limited use because ....

....

....

   Medicine Through Time

Assessment sheet – The introduction of the National Health Service

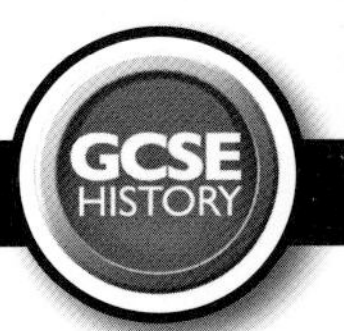

(✓) Tick the boxes to show what you know.

I know:

	know / yes	not sure / sometimes	don't know / no
why the NHS was brought in			
why the Beveridge Report was important			
why many doctors, at first, opposed the NHS			
why the cost of the NHS increased rapidly			
what is meant by the 'nanny state'			
why some people have criticised the NHS			
how to reorganise statements chronologically			
how to explain the utility of a source			
how to explain the limitations of a source			

I know best:

....

I need to work on (up to three targets):

....

....

....

     Medicine Through Time